INFLAMMATORY BOWEL DISEASE

The essential guide to controlling Crohn's Disease, Colitis and other IBDs

Professor John Hunter
MA, MD, FRCP, AGAF

Vermilion
LONDON

1 3 5 7 9 10 8 6 4 2

Published in 2010 by Vermilion, an imprint of Ebury Publishing

Ebury Publishing is a Random House Group company

The Random House Group Limited Reg. No. 954009

Addresses for companies within the Random House Group can be found at
www.rbooks.co.uk

A CIP catalogue record for this book is available from the British Library

The Random House Group Limited supports The Forest Stewardship Council
(FSC), the leading international forest certification organisation. All our titles
that are printed on Greenpeace-approved FSC-certified paper carry the FSC logo.
Our paper procurement policy can be found at
www.rbooks.co.uk/environment

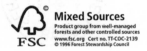

Mixed Sources
Product group from well-managed
forests and other controlled sources
www.fsc.org Cert no. TT-COC-2139
© 1996 Forest Stewardship Council

Printed in Great Britain by Clays Ltd, St Ives plc

ISBN 9780091935085

Copies are available at special rates for bulk orders. Contact the sales
development team on 020 7840 8487 for more information.

To buy books by your favourite authors and register for offers, visit
www.rbooks.co.uk

Contents

Introduction

This book has been written for patients with inflammatory bowel disease (IBD). It is a profound shock to discover that one suffers from a long-lasting disease that produces unpleasant and embarrassing symptoms, may lead to dangerous complications, and for which it is claimed that there is currently no cure. It would be quite wrong, nonetheless, to succumb to pessimism and depression. The aim of this book is to show you how to control these diseases so that you can lead a normal and fulfilling life and enjoy your career, pastimes and family in the same way as your friends and colleagues.

IBD is a complex subject. Even patients with the same diagnosis frequently need quite different treatments. One of my patients with Crohn's disease, a man of 60, had been treated by diet 15 years earlier. His disease had settled well and for the past 10 years he had been on no treatment at all, and in fact had been able to return to a normal diet. He was perplexed when diarrhoea started once again, and wondered if he should go back on his exclusion diet. Investigations, however, showed that his Crohn's disease had burnt itself out, but that the part of the small bowel that had previously been affected was scarred. This meant that it was no longer capable of reabsorbing bile salts and it was these passing into the large intestine that caused his diarrhoea. When given some medication to stop bile salts irritating the large intestine, his diarrhoea ceased and his Crohn's disease remains inactive.

Similarly, it is a common mistake to think that every symptom suffered by a patient with IBD is necessarily caused by the IBD. Another patient of mine, a woman of 45 with Crohn's disease, had severe damage to the small intestine, but this settled beautifully on dietary treatment with an improvement in her X-rays that greatly surprised her local specialist. Her original Crohn's pains and diarrhoea cleared up. However, a few months later she developed further abdominal pains, but in a different place. She was told that this must be further trouble caused by Crohn's disease and her local specialist wanted to put her back on to prednisolone. However, further investigation showed that the new pain was not caused by Crohn's disease at all! The woman had a blockage in her nasal passages that meant that she had started to breathe through her mouth. Because of mouth breathing she was swallowing air, and it was air collecting and distending her stomach that caused her pain. She was sent to see an ear, nose and throat (ENT) surgeon who performed an operation to unblock her nasal airway. When she was able to breathe properly through her nose again, the air swallowing stopped and her pain disappeared. She continues well on her diet with no activity of the Crohn's disease remaining.

Many people have very negative views on IBD. 'We don't know its cause', 'there will be unexpected relapses and remissions', 'you must understand that there is no cure'. It is my belief that recent research has made such dismal Jeremiahs way out of date. We do not know exactly everything perhaps, but we know a very great deal about IBD, and can make intelligent suggestions to fill in the gaps. This knowledge has enabled me to develop a logical and practical approach to IBD that has proved very valuable. Successful treatment should nowadays be seen to be the norm, not the exception. This book is designed to give you the information you need to be an active partner with your health advisors in ensuring that your IBD is kept fully at bay so that you are symptom free and able to live life to the full. No less a goal is acceptable. If IBD is not controlled it may come to dominate your life and considerably curtail your activities. If, however, you understand what is happening to your body and how the disease may be regulated, then you will control the situation and you, and not your IBD, will be the master.

The management of IBD requires great attention to detail. To achieve the best results it is vital that you have a doctor whom you trust. IBD is not a condition to be treated by Do-It-Yourself medicine and you will need treatment and advice that can only be provided by a sympathetic and experienced doctor with a positive outlook on IBD. You must be able to discuss your illness and its problems without embarrassment and you must be confident that your questions and anxieties are falling on receptive ears. Just as there are horses for courses, so there are doctors and patients who get on well together and those who fail to do so! If you are ill at ease with your gastroenterologist get your GP to arrange for you to see someone else.

Nowadays, many hospitals have specialist nurses to help patients with IBD. These too are an invaluable source of knowledge and support whom it is often possible to contact quickly and easily when problems arise.

For your part you must play a full and active role in your disease. Your doctor or nurse cannot be with you 24 hours a day. Throughout your daily activities you must keep a weather eye open to see whether or not they may affect your illness, and discuss with your medical advisors any developments that appear relevant to its control.

Finding you have IBD is a little similar to being suddenly and unexpectedly landed with the care of a very large, ugly and noisy dog, which, if you don't keep it under control, will not only bark incessantly, but will turn round and bite or maul you very painfully when you least expect it. If you train it successfully, though, the horrible dog will sleep quietly in front of the fire, not even stirring to wag its tail. After a few years, if you have kept it well trained and obedient, you will find that it has crept quietly away in the night. Wonderful!

CHAPTER 1

What is inflammatory bowel disease (IBD)?

THE NORMAL HUMAN GUT

The human gut is remarkable. Humans are omnivores – capable of digesting and absorbing nutrients from almost all types of food be they derived from animal or plant sources. We have teeth to enable us to eat meat and a moderately large colon to help digest fibrous fruit and vegetables; we can be perfectly healthy and well nourished on a mixed, balanced diet. This should contain protein – animal proteins are most fully assimilated by the body – carbohydrates and fats as well, of course, as vitamins and minerals.

During a meal food is cut up into smaller pieces by chewing and is mixed with saliva, which not only provides an enzyme to start breaking down carbohydrates but also serves as a lubricant enabling the food to be swallowed easily and pass smoothly down the long tube – the gullet or oesophagus – into the stomach (see fig. 1). Here it stays for one or two hours while it is churned up by contractions of the muscular stomach wall and mixed with acid and further enzymes to speed digestion.

This process makes the food mixture (chyme) liquid. It then passes into the small intestine (see fig. 1) – six to seven metres long – where the process of digestion is completed. The food is broken down by enzymes secreted by the glands of the intestinal wall and by the pancreas. Proteins such as meat, eggs and fish are broken down further and further into short strips of amino acids (peptides) and ultimately to single amino acids themselves. These, together with short strips of amino acids called di- or tripeptides, can be absorbed from the small intestine into the body and serve to build body tissue such as muscle or bone or to be further converted into sugars. Likewise, complex carbohydrate foods such as bread, potatoes and rice are broken down into sugars before absorption. These serve as a major source of energy. Fat digestion is more complex as fat does not dissolve readily in water. Special chemicals, bile salts, are produced in the liver and secreted in the bile. These form little collections called micelles around the fatty molecules. In these micelles fats are digested into fatty acids and glycerol for absorption into the body. After fat digestion is complete, the bile acids are reabsorbed into the body by special cells in the last part of the small intestine, the terminal ileum (see fig. 1) and recycled to the liver. They are secreted into the bile again ready to help digest the next meal.

Some parts of our food – fibre, for example – are not digestible in the small intestine and pass on into the large intestine together with small quantities of carbohydrate and fat that have escaped digestion.

It used to be thought that the large intestine, or colon, (see fig. 1) was relatively unimportant, a mere tube by which waste matter could be channelled out of the body and that its main function in land-dwelling animals such as man was to extract water from the faeces to resist dehydration. This view is now known to be much too simple. In contrast to the small intestine where the digestive enzymes produce an environment that is hostile to bacterial growth and is therefore almost completely sterile, the large intestine contains vast numbers of different bacteria. In each gram of faeces there may be as many as a trillion bacteria comprising over

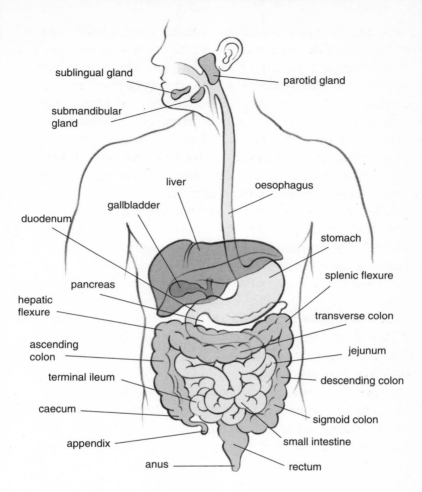

Fig. 1: Diagram of a normal gut

500 strains and species – and the full range is still unknown. Each bacterium contains its own complement of enzymes for digesting and modifying various chemicals so that in combination the bacteria provide a highly complex metabolic system that helps the body deal with a vast range of potentially harmful chemicals taken in from the environment. Of all the body organs, only the liver

(see fig. 1) is more complex in terms of maintaining the body in health. Thus many toxic substances, for example carcinogens (which may promote cancer), are broken down by the bacteria in the large intestine, and beneficial compounds, such as short chain fatty acids used as energy sources by the body, are synthesised, as are vitamins, for example vitamins B and K. We are only now coming to realise that malfunction of the bacteria in the large intestine may underlie a range of important diseases affecting not only the gut but also other parts of the body such as joints and skin and even perhaps the nervous system. These diseases have been called 'enterometabolic' disorders. I believe that one of the most important groups of enterometabolic disorders is IBD.

The obvious result of bacterial action on the undigested food residues coming from the small intestine is, of course, the production of faeces. The residues take perhaps 24 hours to pass through the large intestine and are usually voided daily through the anus. The passage of faeces along the colon is the result of contraction of muscles in the bowel wall over which we have no control, a process known as peristalsis. These muscles work best when the stool is large and soft in texture. Small hard stools proceed with some difficulty. Defecation itself is complex as this is under voluntary control. The anal sphincter, a band of muscle forming a ring round the very lowest part of the bowel, acts as a stopper to prevent leakage. The muscles of the abdominal wall contract and cause the pressure in the abdomen to rise in order to expel the stool, but this by itself would merely push the anus downwards. The muscles of the pelvic floor must contract to pull the anus up, and at the same time the anal sphincter must relax to allow the stool to pass through. The lining of the anus is quite soft and may be torn by hard faecal masses, forming a split known as a fissure-in-ano.

WHAT IS INFLAMMATORY BOWEL DISEASE?

The two most important inflammatory bowel diseases are Crohn's disease (CD) and ulcerative colitis (UC).

UC was at first difficult to distinguish from infectious diarrhoea and dysentery, which were very common before reliable supplies of clean water became available. The first description was probably in 1859, by an Englishman called Wilks. CD was difficult to distinguish from tuberculosis affecting the small intestine, which was also common before pasteurisation of milk was introduced. The first description of CD was by a Scotsman, Dalziel, in 1912, but a clearer account of the condition was published by Burrill Crohn and his colleagues in New York in 1932, and the disease, which they called regional ileitis, subsequently was renamed after him.

UC is a disease in which the large intestine, but not the small, becomes inflamed and ulcerated. In UC it is only the inner lining of the bowel, and not its full thickness, which is affected. UC may affect just the rectum, when it is usually called 'proctitis', or it may affect the bowel from anus to splenic flexure (see fig. 1), when it is referred to as 'left-sided colitis'. If the whole bowel from anus to caecum (see fig. 1) is involved it is called 'pancolitis'. Complications outside the intestine may occur, as in CD, but removing the whole large intestine will cure UC – although the patient will be left with an artificial opening for emptying the bowel, either a stoma or an internal pouch.

CD is a chronic inflammatory disease that can affect the whole of the alimentary tract from the mouth to the anus. The inflammation extends through all areas of the gut wall and is characteristically patchy in distribution, affecting separate areas of the gut and leaving patches of normal tissue in between. This pattern has been called 'skip lesions'. The most commonly affected sites are the ileum and the first part of the large intestine. CD also frequently affects the anus.

If inadequately treated, Crohn's disease progresses over the years. The initial inflammatory phase passes into a phase where strictures are common, and then into a penetrative phase where fistulae between adjacent organs will arise. The more severe the disease, the faster this progression is likely to be.

CD has a number of characteristic features. Its course is often chronic, with periods of remission when patients are symptom free followed by relapses when the disease flares up. Complications outside the intestine (see page 150) are common. This means that CD has a wide range of symptoms as varied as diarrhoea and abdominal pain, a sore red eye or arthritis. Although the presence of skip lesions implies that only part of the gut may be affected by the disease, cutting out the diseased bowel is not a straightforward solution, and sadly there is a strong tendency for CD to reoccur after surgery. Over half the patients who are operated on for CD will subsequently require another operation and if recurrence is looked for carefully with endoscopic checks on the gut, it can be shown that this occurs in 90% of cases. Surgery, then, does not provide an instant cure for CD.

These are the most important forms of IBD. It still is not absolutely clear whether these are two entirely separate diseases, or whether they form the more distinct ends of a spectrum. Certainly there are cases that are sometimes very difficult to classify as either CD or UC as features of both are present, and such cases are usually labelled 'indeterminate colitis' (see page 18). The most important practical distinction is that UC does not affect the small bowel, so that a detection of small bowel inflammation means that a confident diagnosis of CD may be made. The table below shows the main distinguishing features between CD and UC.

MAIN FEATURES DISTINGUISHING UC FROM CD

	CROHN'S DISEASE (CD)	ULCERATIVE COLITIS (UC)
Small bowel	Often affected	Not affected
Large bowel	Skip lesions, patchy inflammation, segments of bowel affected	Continuous involvement from the anus spreading proximally up the large intestine
Abdominal mass	Common	Unusual
Fistulae	Common	Unusual
Depth of inflammation	Deeper penetrating ulcers	Surface layers of mucosa alone are affected
Histology	Granulomas and lymphoid aggregates	Goblet cells depleted of mucus, crypt abscesses, architectural changes
Response to diet	Excellent	Unresponsive

In UC and CD, there is long-standing (chronic) inflammation of the intestinal mucosa – the lining of the gut. This becomes red, inflamed, ulcerated and bleeding.

Such inflammation causes diarrhoea, abdominal pain and, when severe, fever. Other symptoms arise according to the part of the gut that is affected. If there is inflammation in the lower part of the intestine (rectum and sigmoid colon – see fig. 1), there may be blood in the stools, together with mucus and pus. Inflammation so close to the anus leads to the most unpleasant symptom of tenesmus – a continual feeling of having to rush to the lavatory when there is, in fact, little or nothing in the way of stool to be passed.

If the small bowel is inflamed, nutrients may be poorly

absorbed and this may cause weight loss, and in children may interfere with growth.

Sometimes inflammation may penetrate from the bowel lining into the surrounding tissues. This may cause abscesses mainly around the anus, and tracks known as fistulae between the bowel and adjacent organs such as the skin, bladder or vagina. The bowel may become thickened and swollen so that it becomes possible to feel it through the abdominal wall.

Persisting inflammation and scarring can lead to further problems such as anaemia and loss of protein from the blood, which causes tiredness and fatigue. Scarring may lead to narrowing of the bowel (stricture), which may eventually become so tight as to cause a blockage (intestinal obstruction). In a small number of cases, persisting inflammation may lead to the development of cancer.

INDETERMINATE COLITIS

Indeterminate colitis is a condition in which there is inflammation in the large intestine, but none in the small intestine. Although this suggests that it is truly a form of ulcerative colitis, the colonic inflammation may be patchy and the ulcers more like those of Crohn's disease. However, the histology does not show the characteristics of Crohn's disease and at the end of the day, because it is not possible to make a definite diagnosis of either UC or CD, we call it 'indeterminate colitis'.

This may, however, lead to a lot of confusion. Although the biopsy changes are not definitely diagnostic of CD, they may be suggestive of it, and frequently pathologists will report that the changes are 'consistent' with CD. This often means that the clinicians reading the report jump on

---

the magic words and tell the patient that he is suffering from CD.

I believe that this is the reason that many gastroenterologists claim that diet is not effective in colonic CD. I have seen many patients with classical changes of CD in the large bowel who have responded very well to dietary treatment and enjoyed long remissions. On the other hand there have been patients who have initially seemed to improve on elemental diet (see pages 36 and 91) but relapsed at a later stage and then, unlike CD, failed to respond to a second course. The subsequent reinvestigation of this group of patients usually reveals characteristic changes of UC.

My view, therefore, is that an indeterminate colitis is indeed halfway between UC and CD. I would suggest that in indeterminate colitis the bacteria of the bowel live partly on food residues but are also capable of switching over to get energy from other bowel contents such as mucus. Because the bacteria have been living partly on food residues, the initial course of elemental diet leads to improvement. When they are deprived of the foods they need, however, they switch over to other sources of energy, the immune attack on the bacteria resumes and the patient relapses.

Indeterminate colitis thus presents a difficult problem for clinicians. In my opinion, the presence of small bowel involvement or granulomas (i.e. nodules of cells surrounded by lymphocytes) in biopsies from the large bowel is clear evidence of CD and we can expect over 90% of cases to respond successfully to diet. In cases where only the colon is involved and no granulomas are present, even though the changes may resemble CD, the outlook for dietary treatment is uncertain. There is no harm in trying it, but the response may be disappointing.

OTHER CAUSES OF INFLAMMATION OF THE INTESTINE

There are many reasons why a bowel may become inflamed, and these should be ruled out before a confident diagnosis of UC or CD can be made. The commonest is infection. Many microbes may invade the gut and cause acute inflammation, particularly in hot countries where sanitation is poor.

Usually infections are short-lived and settle after a few days' treatment, but some such as tuberculosis or amoebiasis may become persistent problems. Even short-term infections may be important in the management of patients with IBD as the symptoms produced by an infection may be mistaken for a relapse of IBD and thus treated inappropriately. The damage to the mucosa caused by the infection may appear very similar to that caused by UC or CD. However, infections are readily identified by microscopic examination of the stool for eggs and parasites and by culture for pathogenic bacteria. Such examinations must always be performed when patients with IBD develop recurrent symptoms or appear to relapse.

OTHER FORMS OF COLITIS

MICROSCOPIC COLITIS

Sometimes patients with chronic diarrhoea are found at endoscopy to have no visible inflammation in the intestinal mucosa, but inflammatory changes are present when biopsies are examined under the microscope. Sometimes these changes are typical of CD or UC and a confident diagnosis can be made, but frequently there is inflammation which is not specific and that patient is diagnosed as suffering from microscopic colitis. There are three main groups of micro-scopic colitis:

> **Lymphocytic colitis:** an excess of lymphocytes in the mucosa. Patients usually suffer watery diarrhoea with little blood in the stools.

> **Collagenous colitis:** a band of collagen is seen lying beneath the epithelium as well as chronic inflammation. As in lymphocytic colitis, watery diarrhoea is the predominant symptom.

> **Eosinophilic colitis:** in this there are many eosinophils (cells which are seen to have taken up a red dye when examined under the microscope) lying in the mucosa. The eosinophils are important in parasitic diseases. Patients often have other evidence of allergy such as hay fever or asthma and parasitic infection must always be excluded.

COLITIS ARISING FROM DISEASES ELSEWHERE IN THE BODY

Some diseases which primarily affect other organs may also involve the large intestine.

> **Behçets:** this causes ulcers in the mouth and on the genitals, together with inflammation in the eyes, skin and nervous system. It may cause ulceration in the ileum and caecum, which is very like that seen in CD.

> **Ischaemic colitis:** inflammation of the bowel may arise if the blood supply to the gut is impaired. This is not common as the intestine is richly supplied with blood vessels. It occurs mainly in older

patients who may also have evidence of an impaired blood supply to the heart, nervous system or limbs, but it is also sometimes seen in younger patients who suffer from Hughes syndrome (anti-phospholipid syndrome) where the blood is 'sticky' and may clot more easily, disturbing flow.

⟩ **Radiation colitis:** Inflammation of the intestine may follow radiotherapy for cancer. This may come on sometimes many years after treatment has been completed.

I hope that this book will give you the information and insight into IBD that will enable you to work sensibly and straightforwardly with your doctor and his team so that your IBD is fully controlled and you are able to lead a full, happy and productive life. Understanding your problems is the first step to getting them completely under control!

CHAPTER 2

What is the cause of IBD?

The best way to prevent a disease and to control it is to understand its cause. Unfortunately, a full explanation of the causes of IBD still eludes us despite many years of intense investigation. In this section I shall concentrate attention on those factors believed to be involved in the cause of IBD, which are well established and of practical value in understanding its treatment.

GENETICS

IBD is known to be more frequent in certain groups of individuals – for example, the Jewish race and the Chaldeans, a group living near Detroit in the USA who originally came from Iraq. It is also clear that IBD tends to run in families, indeed first-degree relatives (i.e. parents, siblings and children) of patients with CD have approximately a 1 in 10 chance of developing the disease, compared to 1 in 10,000 of the general population. This is in no way a reason to suggest that it is undesirable for people with CD to have children – an incidence of 1 in 10 means that 90% of relatives will *not* be affected.

It is now known that IBD is not totally genetically determined, as are, for example, colour blindness in boys or haemophilia. Rather, there exist a number of genes that when present *may* increase the likelihood of someone developing IBD. So many different genes are now implicated that the situation has become very complex.

Fig. 2 summarises our current knowledge of the situation. Some genes increase susceptibility to CD, some to UC and some may be important in both conditions.

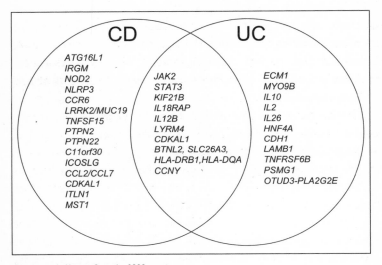

CD | UC

ATG16L1		
IRGM		ECM1
NOD2	JAK2	MYO9B
NLRP3	STAT3	IL10
CCR6	KIF21B	IL2
LRRK2/MUC19	IL18RAP	IL26
TNFSF15	IL12B	HNF4A
PTPN2	LYRM4	CDH1
PTPN22	CDKAL1	LAMB1
C11orf30	BTNL2, SLC26A3,	TNFRSF6B
ICOSLG	HLA-DRB1,HLA-DQA	PSMG1
CCL2/CCL7	CCNY	OTUD3-PLA2G2E
CDKAL1		
ITLN1		
MST1		

Barrett et al. *Nature Genetics* 2008
Fisher SA et al. *Nature Genetics* 2008
Anderson C et al. *Gastroenterology* 2008
W TCCC *Nature Genetics* 2009

Fig. 2: Genetics of inflammatory bowel disease

So many different genes are involved that it is very unlikely that we shall ever be able to control IBD by gene therapy – even if that were a practical possibility. However, some researchers hope that knowledge of a patient's genotype may possibly be of value in determining which treatment for his IBD will prove most suitable. Advances in this field are rapid and complicated!

IMMUNITY

Pathological examination of specimens of bowel removed at surgery from patients with IBD reveals the presence of acute inflammation. These changes are known to result from the release of a complex series of chemicals by the body's immune system. The crucial importance of the immune system in the pathogenesis of IBD has been demonstrated by AIDS. AIDS leads to immune deficiency, knocking out certain lymphocytes – and, interestingly, patients with AIDS who previously had CD find that the CD gets better!

The immune system is of key importance in the protection of the body against infection and disease. At birth, the immune system is not developed and the infant is protected by antibodies passed on by the mother both in the uterus and later in breast milk. During the first three months after birth the immune system comes to recognise all the constituents of the body as 'self' and therefore does not attack them. While a baby is in the uterus, the bowel contains no bacteria. After birth, however, the bacteria colonise the gut, and those entering the bowel in the first weeks of life are also classified by the immune system as 'self' and are not attacked by it. This phenomenon is known as immune tolerance.

Immune tolerance ends after about three months of life. Thereafter all foreign substances – be they invading microbes or transplanted organs such as a kidney – are attacked by the immune system. Such foreign substances are known as antigens and may be the objects of attack by chemicals directed specifically against them called antibodies, or by inflammatory cells such as leucocytes or lymphocytes which may engulf bacteria to destroy them or produce chemicals known as cytokines which protect the body by producing inflammation. As a child matures, he or she develops a wide range of antibodies directed against specific infections to diseases, together with lymphocytes programmed against the antigens that have been encountered. The antibodies are found in the blood amongst a group of chemicals called immunoglobulins. Lymphocytes are found in high numbers in the wall of the gut, where they are ideally positioned to recognise and attack any dangerous microbes present in the food. When these are encountered the release of inflammatory chemicals has the effect of allowing blood to enter the tissue affected, but preventing its release. This increases the concentration of immune cells available to destroy the invading microbes. The tissue becomes red and swollen until the area has been cleared.

In health the immune system only attacks invading microbes and leaves the normal bacteria of the bowel in peace. In IBD, for reasons still uncertain, these friendly bacteria become the objects of immune attack.

This was first shown in 1995 by some German researchers who isolated immune cells from patients with CD. They took the cells both from the blood and also from the lining of the gut in areas where inflammation was active and in others where it was not. They then tested to see whether or not these cells would mount an immune attack on bacteria which they had either taken from the same patient whose immune cells were being tested, or from another person completely. As might be expected, all the cells reacted to foreign bacteria taken from another person and failed to respond to bacteria taken from the same patient that they themselves had come from. The only exception to this was that immune cells from areas of the intestine where there was active CD reacted just as vigorously to bacteria from their host patient in just the same way as they did to react to bacteria from others. In other words, these cells were attacking their own 'home' bacteria. Thus the immune tolerance to the host bacteria normally present from birth had been broken.

We were able to support this finding by looking at the same problem from another angle. We took faeces from patients with active IBD and determined how many bacteria were being attacked by the immune system by measuring the percentage of bacteria coated by the patients' antibodies (immunoglobulins). Normally only about 20% of bacteria are so affected. These probably represent foreign bacteria, whether harmful or not, which have been swallowed and are passing through the gut. In our patients with IBD, however, as much as 80–90% of bacteria were coated with immunoglobulin. Further, after only two weeks' treatment with prednisolone (page 130) for UC or elemental diet for CD, the percentage of coated bacteria fell significantly. Other patients, whether suffering from UC or CD, who had been in remission for at least two years, had normal levels of coated bacteria – back to 20%. Thus an immune attack on the resident bacteria of the intestine is a key factor in causing IBD. Why the usual immune tolerance breaks down is not clear. It is well known that other conditions may arise in which the body attacks its own tissues. Two well-known examples are Hashimoto's disease, where the body produces antibodies which eventually destroy the thyroid gland and lupus where antibodies directed against the nuclei of the body's cells may set up inflammation in different organs such as the kidneys or the skin. In UC and CD, circulating antibodies have been discovered that are indeed directed against the bacteria of the gut, but unlike Hashimoto's disease and lupus, where detection of antibodies is an important diagnostic tool, antibody tests are of little value in the diagnosis of IBD.

Thus the immune system plays a central role in producing IBD and this has been reflected in its treatment. As we shall see later, a key part of the treatment of IBD involves reducing the activity of the immune system. This can involve reducing its overall activity by such drugs as corticosteroids or azathioprine, by blocking specific cytokines such as TNF-α by infliximab or even by removing immune cells by a process known as plasmapheresis.

It has even been possible to trick the immune system. The classic immune response leading to inflammation is called a Th1 response and this is what occurs in IBD, especially in CD. The immune response to worm infestations and allergy is called Th2. If a Th2 response can be provoked, Th1 responses may be reduced. Thus some workers have been able to reduce inflammation in CD by the administration of eggs of harmless worms, such as *Trichuris suis*, derived from pigs. Patients given these worms certainly improve in the short term, but how long this remission is maintained remains to be seen.

BACTERIA

It is well recognised that the onset of IBD, whether UC or Crohn's, may follow bacterial infections such as gastroenteritis. One of my patients was perfectly well until he was 16 when he went off to camp with five or six members of his scout patrol. Perhaps none of them had gained their hygiene or food handlers' badges as the whole patrol came down with a nasty bout of gastroenteritis and had to return home several days prematurely. Over the next few days all the members of the patrol recovered fully with the exception of one – my patient, whose diarrhoea continued for several weeks and who, when he was referred to hospital, proved to have developed UC. He obviously had genetic susceptibility to IBD – perhaps his fellow scouts didn't!

IBD may therefore follow a bout of gastrointestinal infection, which may also trigger relapses in patients who have been in long-term remission. There is also an increased frequency of onset or relapse of IBD after courses of anti-biotics, which may also damage the bacteria of the bowel.

It is unsurprising therefore that many have suggested that IBD is the result of a microbial infection and that possibly a definite organism may be responsible. Several bacteria have been proposed as possible causes, but none has yet proved convincing.

ENTEROPATHIC *ESCHERICIA COLI*

E. coli is the bacterium that may cause gastroenteritis. It carries an antigen which is also found in the lining of the bowel. Some years ago there was great excitement that an antibody to this antigen might be produced after being infected with *E. coli*, which could conceivably continue to cause inflammation in the bowel lining when the infection had passed. Furthermore, in as many as 65% of cases of CD, these bacteria were found to be adherent to the small bowel mucosa. However, later research has suggested that neither these antibodies nor the adherent bacteria have the capacity to cause tissue damage and thus lead to disease.

MEASLES

The possible role of MMR (Measles, Mumps and Rubella) immunisation in causing CD has raised such controversy as to spill into the national press and lead to eminent gastroenterologists appearing before the General Medical Council. Chronic infection with measles and related paramyxoviruses may indeed lead to chronic human disease particularly of the nervous system, but there is now no support for the role of the organisms in IBD and children must not be denied MMR immunisation for this reason.

SULPHATE-REDUCING BACTERIA

Bacterial fermentation of food residues in the large intestine leads to the production of vast quantities of hydrogen that must be eliminated. This is usually done by bacteria, which convert it into methane, but in some people bacteria called sulphate-reducing bacteria (SRBs) help to dispose of it by using it to convert sulphate to hydrogen sulphide. This gas is well known to schoolchildren in chemistry laboratories for smelling of 'bad eggs'. Many patients with colitis complain that their rectal flatus becomes offensive. It has been shown that stools in patients with UC produce as much as four times more hydrogen sulphide than those of healthy persons. What is more, hydrogen sulphide is very poisonous and it has been suggested that its excess production could therefore lead to the development of inflammation of the large bowel.

However, it has not been possible to demonstrate any great number or activity of SRBs in patients with UC than in the normal population. Nor have attempts to treat UC by reducing the amount of sulphate in the diet in the hope of reducing hydrogen sulphide production proved successful. It seems unlikely that SRBs themselves can be the cause of UC. Nevertheless, sulphur metabolism may still prove to be very important. In experiments nearly 100 years ago it was shown that hydrogen sulphide was very poisonous to dogs when given by mouth. However, when the same amount was administered by an enema into the large intestine, the dogs survived, but the amount of sulphate in the blood increased. This suggests that the bacteria of the bowel can reconvert hydrogen sulphide to sulphate, preventing toxic amounts of the gas accumulating. It is possible that interference with this recycling of hydrogen sulphide may be an important factor in producing inflammation in UC.

FAECALIBACTERIUM PRAUSNITZII (FP)

The presence of a specific pathogen such as salmonella or shigella is one way in which a microbe may cause disease. It has also been suggested than an alternative mechanism for the cause of CD could be the loss from the body of a protective microbe that prevented inflammation. Some French researchers recently cultured bacteria from samples of intestine removed from patients with CD at surgery and showed that very low numbers of an organism called *Faecalibacterium prausnitzii* were present. They also showed that chemicals derived from this microbe had an anti-inflammatory effect raising hopes that CD might be treatable by restoring the numbers of Fp in the bowel to normal levels.

We recently tried to confirm this work by searching for Fp in patients with CD, UC and irritable bowel syndrome (IBS), as well as healthy controls. Our work differed from that of the French group in that we studied faeces rather than surgical specimens. The composition of faeces may alter as it passes along the bowel. We found no difference at all in the numbers of Fp in our all groups – the levels in CD were little less than in our normal controls. Furthermore, when our CD patients were treated with elemental diet (pages 36, 91), the numbers of Fp in the faeces fell. Indeed there was a significant correlation: the better the response to treatment the greater the fall in Fp numbers. It therefore seems unlikely that Fp is an important factor in preventing CD.

MYCOBACTERIUM PARATUBERCULOSIS (MAP)

This bacterium is closely related to the organism that causes tuberculosis and is known to cause a disease of the intestine in cattle called Johne's disease. MAP is widespread in the environment in Britain and is not destroyed by pasteurisation of cows' milk. It causes infection in immunosuppressed patients, such as those suffering from AIDS. The changes in the bowel in Johne's disease resemble in some ways those seen in CD and it has therefore been suggested that MAP might be the cause of both conditions.

Support for this suggestion was provided by the isolation of MAP, both as bacterial DNA and as intact organisms, from many more cases of CD than from other gut diseases. However, this does not necessarily mean that MAP causes the disease; it could equally be true that MAP was present merely as a secondary contaminant in tissue already severely damaged by CD. The epidemiological evidence is against an important role for MAP, as CD is no more frequent in vets and farmers than in the general population, despite their greater exposure to cattle with Johne's disease. Furthermore, although there has been no case of Johne's disease in Sweden for the last 30 years, the incidence of CD has increased there just as it has in the rest of northern Europe.

The T-spot test is widely used to diagnose tuberculosis. It detects lymphocytes circulating in the blood of patients that are targeted against antigens in the tubercle bacterium. We used this test to look for lymphocytes targeted against MAP in CD with negative results.

Reports exist of improvement in CD when patients were treated by antibiotics effective against MAP, but these drugs are nonspecific in their effects and many will attack other bacteria as well (see page 88). On balance, it is improbable that MAP causes CD.

THE NORMAL GASTROINTESTINAL BACTERIA AS A CAUSE OF IBD

The famous 19th-century German microbiologist Robert Koch enunciated postulates to show that a microbe caused disease:

1. It should be present in every case of the disease occurring in the primary host

2. When isolated from the diseased primary host, the organism should be able to be grown in a secondary host

3. When the organism is taken from the secondary host it would still cause the disease in the primary host

None of the bacteria so far suggested to cause IBD fulfil these postulates.

This does not mean that a specific microbe which causes IBD may not still be discovered. We now know that *Helicobacter pylori* is an important cause of gastritis and duodenal ulcers, but this bacterium was not able to be grown until 1983. Before then it was thought that duodenal ulcers were largely caused by stress; since *Helicobacter pylori* was discovered and the means of eliminating it established, ulcers have virtually disappeared – even in workaholics!

In a recent study of the gut bacteria in CD, only 60% of the organisms present could be accurately characterised and identified. There is still the possibility that an unknown bacterium – perhaps '*Helicobacter crohnsii*' – may be lurking amongst the remaining 30–40% of bacteria of which we know so little!

It appears more likely perhaps that the link between UC and CD and the gut bacteria represents not the effect of a single pathogen, but of a loss of tolerance to the normal intestinal bacteria. We know that anything that reduces the number of bacteria in the bowel – be it washing out the intestine with enemas or purges, antibiotics, creation of an ileostomy or intravenous feeding – may produce therapeutic benefit. An elegant study by Belgian researchers showed the importance of the intestinal fluid in producing CD. They studied patients who had undergone surgery with the removal of the damaged bowel so that the end of the small bowel was then rejoined (anastamosed) to the large intestine. To allow the anastamosis to heal easily a temporary ileostomy was performed higher up so that all the intestinal fluid passed out of the body without reaching the anastamosis. Colonoscopy at this stage revealed the bowel below the ileostomy to be quite healthy. The ileostomy was then removed so that the intestinal fluid passed along the bowel again and through the anastamosis. Further colonoscopies six months later showed that the CD had returned in every case.

Of all the components of the intestinal fluid – food residues, intestinal secretions and bacteria – food and bacteria are the most likely agents to provoke disease. The role of food and diet is discussed later (page 35). But it seems unlikely that food itself is the main culprit. The finger of suspicion points firmly at the gut bacteria.

Although we have so far been unable to detect a specific pathogen, we can only identify accurately two-thirds of the bacteria living in the gut in IBD. Nevertheless, despite this handicap we know that the resident flora in IBD is different from that in healthy individuals. In particular, there is an increase in organisms that normally would prefer to grow in the presence of oxygen. The large bowel contains very little oxygen under normal circumstances and in health, not surprisingly, there are relatively few of the oxygen-loving bacteria (aerobes) present. Each gram of faeces contains about 1 trillion bacteria. In health only 100,000 of these are aerobes. In IBD the number of aerobes may increase by as much as 100,000 to reach a figure as high as 10 billion. Perhaps this may lead to a profound change in the processes of bacterial fermentation in the bowel provoking an immune response against the bacteria concerned and that this is what leads to disease. This possibility is now under vigorous investigation. Nevertheless, it cannot be the whole explanation. Similar changes in the bacterial flora are seen in IBS where there is little if any inflammation of the gastrointestinal mucosa. It may be that genetic factors influence the intestinal response to changes in bacterial metabolism. It has recently been suggested, for example, that increased permeability of the lining of the intestine may be increased not only in patients with CD but also in their relatives suggesting it might be under genetic control. This might allow bacteria to penetrate to deeper levels of the intestinal wall where an immunological attack could lead to tissue inflammation and disease.

DIET

All patients with IBD and many of their doctors have wondered whether diet might be one of the causes of their illness. The dramatic successes following gluten-free diets for coeliac disease and exclusion diets for the management of IBS have inevitably heightened such speculation.

In 1976 some German physicians reported that children suffering from CD ate large quantities of sweets. Despite difficulties with methodology, a number of subsequent studies confirmed that the diets of patients with CD were indeed different, with increased intake not only of sugar, but also of cornflakes. Likewise, a prospective epidemiological study in Japan demonstrated a strong correlation between the incidence of CD and the consumption of fat, with reduction in omega-3 and increased omega-6 fatty acids of particular importance. A recent study from Norfolk has suggested that eating more than 30g of oleic acid (from olive oil) daily may reduce the risk of developing UC in the elderly.

However, there is as yet no evidence that modifying the diet in this way is of therapeutic benefit in established IBD. A prospective multicentre British trial designed to assess the value of a high-residue diet low in sugar and prepared foods showed no benefit in CD and it is now clear that the real reason that CD patients eat extra amounts of foods rich in sugar is because they relieve hunger and provide

---

THE ELEMENTAL DIET

Elemental diets are liquid feeds which are pre-digested, so that instead of starches they contain sugars and instead of proteins, amino acids or peptides. A single fat source is added, together with vitamins and minerals to make them nutritionally complete.

Elemental feeds are further classified according to the way in which nitrogen (from protein) is presented. A true elemental feed contains nitrogen in the form of amino acids alone; some, however, contain it as short chains of linked amino acids (di- and tripeptides) and these are known as oligomeric. Polymeric feeds contain nitrogen as a single whole protein. Whey from cows' milk is a typical example.

---

energy while provoking fewer symptoms and causing less discomfort.

Further interest in the possible role of diet followed reports of improvement in patients with CD (but not UC) after both parenteral and enteral feeding. Total parenteral nutrition (TPN) is potentially dangerous and expensive and is nowadays little used for uncomplicated CD. Enteral feeds, on the other hand, whether elemental or polymeric, are clearly highly effective at inducing remission when used as the sole source of nutrition for two to three weeks. Not only do patients go into symptomatic remission, but objective blood tests such as sedimentation rate, serum C-reactive protein and albumin concentrations return to normal and the mucosa heals. Unfortunately, as many as one-third of patients are unable or unwilling to comply with such a long period of enteral feeding and this inevitably reduces the overall success rate. However, the success rates in those patients who do complete the course of feeding is 80%–90%, a figure comfortably in excess of any other therapy for CD currently available.

PARENTERAL VS ENTERAL FEEDING

parenteral feeding: *where the patient receives nutrition through the veins.*

enteral feeding: *where the patient receives nutrition as a liquid feed, often of special composition, which may be taken by mouth, or sometimes through the nose via a naso-gastric tube or directly into the stomach through the abdominal wall via a percutaneous endoscopic gastrostomy (PEG).*

Subsequent reintroduction of foods, one by one, allows identification of any that provoke symptoms. The food intolerances reported by patients receiving nutritional therapy for CD vary widely. The most common are gluten, corn, dairy products and yeast, but others may be as disparate as chocolate, pork and onions. The wide range of intolerances reported by different patients make it unlikely that the foods themselves cause the disease. What, then, is the mechanism by which enteral feeds induce remission?

RAST or skin-prick testing reveals no evidence of IgE- (immunoglobin E-) mediated food allergy, and the incidence of allergy in CD is no greater than that in the general population. Simple improvement of nutrition seems unlikely as a reduction in inflammatory markers can be clearly detected before there is any sign of nutritional improvement. It is unlikely that elemental diet can have any intrinsic anti-inflammatory effect itself, as it is known to be ineffective in UC. The early suggestion that it induced 'bowel rest' has been abandoned, since it was shown that enteral feeding had a therapeutic effect even when patients were eating normal foodstuffs as well.

A similar food intolerance to that reported in CD has also been demonstrated by double-blind testing in some patients with IBS. Hydrogen and methane production in newly diagnosed cases of IBS were measured in a calorimeter. The total hydrogen production and maximal excretion rate were significantly reduced as were symptoms in the patients, but not in healthy controls, after two weeks on an exclusion diet avoiding those foods known to be most likely to provoke symptoms in IBS. Similar effects were produced by antibiotics and a diet that avoids fibre completely. Since hydrogen cannot be produced by the mammalian cell, these studies provided strong evidence that the metabolic activity of colonic bacteria lay at the root of symptoms in some cases of IBS.

A similar mechanism may exist in CD. As we have seen, the colonic bacterial flora is abnormal in CD. Circumstantial evidence for a change in the activity of colonic bacteria comes from the observations that the stools turn green in patients on enteral feeds (because of reduction in bacterial conversion of biliverdin to stercobilin) and that breath odour becomes unpleasant (because chemicals normally broken down by bacteria in the colon are released on the breath). Perhaps the most striking evidence in support of this theory so far is that 80%–100% of colonic bacteria in patients with active CD are coated with immunoglobulin, compared to 20% in controls and in IBD in remission. Significant falls in the number of organisms coated with IgG (immunoglobin G) or IgM (immunoglobin M) occur after two weeks of enteral feeding with elemental diet in CD and a similar length of corticosteroid treatment in UC.

This suggests that the immune response in CD is directed against the host faecal flora, and that depriving the flora of its nutritional substrates by enteral feeding significantly reduces the immune response directed against it. It seems probable that food itself is not a factor in the pathogenesis of CD, but that food residues that promote the metabolic activity of an abnormal intestinal microflora may allow the disease to progress.

SMOKING

The risk of developing IBD has not been shown to be linked to alcohol consumption. There is now clear evidence, however, that smoking affects IBD, but in different ways in CD and UC. Stopping smoking after a diagnosis of CD reduces the likelihood of surgery and prolongs the length of remission. The relapse rate per year is reduced by 40%.

Clearly patients with CD should not smoke. This is discussed in detail in chapter 9.

By contrast, smokers are less likely to suffer from UC and indeed the highest frequency of UC in a study in South Wales was in those who had *stopped* smoking. The benefits of smoking in UC, however, are far outweighed by the other risks to smokers such as heart disease, chronic bronchitis and cancer.

The reason for the effect of smoking in IBD is still uncertain. Nicotine is, of course, an important constituent of cigarette smoke, but attempts to treat UC with nicotine patches have only proved modestly successful. I personally believe that the beneficial effect of smoking in UC is due to its well-known mild laxative effect, which relieves problems such as mild proximal constipation (see page 146).

The effect of smoking on intestinal mucus and the function of white cells may possibly be important, but the full mechanism remains to be sorted out. The simple message, however, is that all patients with IBD should avoid smoking.

ANTI-INFLAMMATORY DRUGS

Non-steroidal anti-inflammatory drugs (NSAIDs) have been implicated as a factor causing some cases of IBD. Examples are aspirin, diclofenac and ibuprofen, and a full list is given in the table below. These drugs are used very frequently in patients with arthritis to reduce joint pain and swelling by blocking the production of inflammatory prostaglandins. They also block the production of prostaglandins, which are important in the defences of the gut. This leads to increased intestinal permeability and allows bacterial penetration through the mucosa. White-cell studies (see page 62) have shown small bowel ulceration in patients taking NSAIDs for arthritis which persisted for as much as a year after treatment had been stopped.

NSAIDs may cause watery diarrhoea and chronic blood loss. These effects may be worse in patients with IBD where they should of course be avoided as far as possible.

ANTI-INFLAMMATORY DRUGS THAT MAY UPSET IBD	
Aceclofenac (Preservex)	Ibuprofen (Brufen, Fenbid, Nurofen)
Acemetacin (Emflex)	
Aspirin (many preparations – check on packet)	Indometacin (Indomethacin, Flexin Continus)
Celecoxib (Celebrex)	Ketoprofen (Orudis, Orovail)
Dexibuprofen (Seractil)	Lumiracoxib (Prexige)
Dexketoprofen (Keral)	Mefenamic Acid (Ponstan)
Diclofenac Sodium (Voltarol, Diclomax, Arthrotec)	Meloxicam (Mobic)
	Nabumetone (Relifex)
Diflunisal (Dolobid)	Naproxen (Naprosyn, Synflex, Napratec)
Etodolac (Lodine)	
Etoricoxib (Arcoxia)	Piroxicam (Brexidol, Feldene)
Fenbufen (Lederfen)	Sulindac (Clinoril)
Fenoprofen (Fenopron)	Tenoxicam (Mobiflex)
Flurbiprofen (Froben)	Tiaprofenic Acid (Surgam)

SEX HORMONES

IBD is predominantly a disease of puberty. It's rare in the under-tens and the peak incidence is in the second and third decades. Although the prevalence in men and women is much the same, older patients affected are much more likely to be men and so it follows that it is women who are most likely to be affected during the reproductive years. There is a frequent variation of symptoms of IBD from phase to phase of the menstrual cycle and the behaviour in IBD changes in pregnancy (see page 219). Thus the importance of female sex hormones in IBD becomes apparent.

The reason for this could be the effect of sex hormones, particularly progesterone, on the metabolic activity of the intestinal bacteria. Some researchers believed that they had discovered a new sex hormone when they identified a chemical in the urine of women that increased just before their periods. Further analysis revealed that the chemical was derived from lignans, a substance found in the cellulose which makes up the walls of plant cells. The breakdown of lignans was being carried out by the bacteria in the gut; when the women were given an antibiotic that stopped bacterial activity, the new chemical disappeared from the urine. Thus, there was no new sex hormone – but clear evidence that bacterial activity was influenced by the hormones of the menstrual cycle.

PSYCHOLOGICAL FACTORS

Patients with IBD that has been poorly controlled and who have suffered persistent abdominal pain and urgent diarrhoea with little relief often become anxious and depressed. To an observer, such psychological changes may appear more obvious than the actual gut symptoms themselves, for people are naturally very reticent in discussing bowel upsets and belly aches. It's common knowledge that our bowels may become loose when we are stressed, for example, before an exam or a big sporting event. It's not surprising therefore that some physicians have suggested that IBD may be a psychosomatic disorder – that is to say, that the bowel symptoms are the results of mental turmoil. Indeed, one well-known East Anglian physician used to play recordings of the voices of his patients claiming that he could differentiate between UC and CD by the tenor of their voices and the stresses which this demonstrated.

Our current detailed knowledge of the inflammatory changes seen in IBD has made such a view untenable. We no longer believe that IBD is 'all in the mind'.

Nevertheless it is well recognised that a flare of IBD may follow stressful events. One young patient of mine had UC, which was so well controlled that she had stopped taking any treatment. One day while out shopping a piece of metal fell on her head from some scaffolding she passed by, causing a nasty cut. She was greatly shocked and distressed. Three days later her UC relapsed and took several months of treatment to bring it back under control. It was difficult not to believe that the stress had not led to this relapse. Many physicians have reported similar occurrences.

Psychological factors do not cause IBD, therefore, but they certainly may make it worse. The reasons for this are still unknown. My personal belief is that one of the effects of stress is an abnormal breathing pattern called over-breathing. Over-breathing increases the amount of air that we swallow. This may pass down the gut and reach the large intestine. As it contains 20% of oxygen, such swallowed air may promote the growth of the oxygen-loving bacteria whose numbers, as we have discussed, are increased in IBD. Increased activity of these microbes might possibly lead to a relapse. However, this theory remains to be investigated.

SUMMARY AND CONCLUSIONS

The cause of IBD is still not fully understood. In the preceding account I have tried to simplify a hugely complex topic.

I freely admit to having ignored much material that many of my fellow gastroenterologists would consider of great importance, but which I have judged to be either confusing or irrelevant. My aim has been to provide you with a fairly simple model that will help you understand IBD and its management. For this I make no apology.

IBD arises as a result of an increase of the metabolic activity of the bacteria in the gastrointestinal tract. This may be initiated by gastrointestinal infection, or antibiotics and possibly by other as yet unknown causes. In genetically susceptible persons, such factors provoke an attack by the body's immune system on the bacteria leading to inflammation of the gut mucosa. This attack may be modified by other factors – bacterial activity, for example, by diet and female sex hormones and possibly also by stress. The immune response may be affected by other diseases such as AIDS or worm infestations and the effect on the bowel tissues themselves may be modified by factors affecting their defences, such as smoking and non-steroidal anti-inflammatory drugs.

Keep this model in mind and we shall proceed to use it to help us plan the logical management of IBD.

CHAPTER 3

Symptoms of IBD

The diagnosis of IBD is often not straightforward. It is not unusual for some months to elapse between the first symptoms and the establishment of a definite diagnosis. This is because the predominant symptoms of IBD – diarrhoea, abdominal pain, weight loss and fatigue – are also produced by many other disorders.

One young woman referred to me was an inpatient at a neighbouring psychiatric hospital. She had been admitted there because she was thought to have anorexia nervosa – the so-called 'slimmer's disease'. Her weight was continuing to fall despite her psychiatrist's best efforts and I was asked to supply specialist nutritional support in order to prevent this. She had no diarrhoea or abdominal pain. However, investigation at Addenbrooke's revealed the presence of inflammation in the blood, and X-rays confirmed the presence of CD in the small intestine. When started on elemental diet the patient rapidly regained weight and made a full recovery without the need for any further psychiatric treatment. Patients with suspected anorexia must always be investigated to make sure they don't have CD.

Even when a patient has symptoms more obviously focused on the gut, it must be appreciated that there is a number of other disorders that produce diarrhoea and abdominal pain that are far more common than IBD. In this chapter I will put the symptoms of IBD in perspective. This will help you to understand the other possibilities that your doctor will consider as he weighs up your case, and show you how to describe your symptoms more clearly. We shall also go through a range of symptoms that might seem apparently unrelated to IBD, but which may be important pointers to its presence. Do not forget to check these out and let your doctor know if they apply to you!

Many of the symptoms of IBD are very embarrassing. People don't like talking about their bowels. I remember once as a very young doctor being at a posh dinner and being asked by a patronising neighbour what had been my most difficult experience as a medical student. I told him, truthfully, that it had been having to ask a man old enough to be my father about his bowels. My neighbour snorted, and then, without replying, turned away and refused to speak to me for the rest of the evening! But doctors grow older and become hardened, and gastroenterologists in particular have heard it all. You won't embarrass your doctor by telling him your diarrhoea is so bad that you have had an accident – so don't let it embarrass you! It is in everyone's interest for you to give your doctors a complete and accurate picture of your symptoms – yours, because it will mean the doctor takes your problem seriously, and his or hers, because a clear picture of the problem emerges, which is an enormous help in diagnosis. If you really feel that you can no more describe your symptoms completely than you could talk about sex to your grandmother, then write everything down, and let the doctor read it!

COMMON CAUSES OF DIARRHOEA

Diarrhoea is a word that means different things to different people. Medical purists often claim that the only reliable way to decide whether someone has diarrhoea or not is to weigh the patient's stools. Ideal for research, perhaps, but hardly suitable for everyday use! In general, most people use the word to describe stools that are frequent, loose, or both. Few healthy people have their bowels open more than three times a day, or less often than once every three days. Stools may be loose – especially after a good party or a hot curry – but if you only go once or twice, it doesn't really count as diarrhoea.

An important feature of diarrhoea is urgency – the need to dash to the loo without any delay. It may help to gauge the severity of the problem if you think to yourself how long you can wait before you have to dash. Minutes? Seconds? Do you have to stop the car and dive behind a hedge? Do you ever have an accident? Before you see your doctor, try to count up the number of times you have passed a motion in the previous 24 hours. This figure will be of great help to your doctor in deciding how severe the problem may be.

Infections are the most common cause of severe diarrhoea. These may be caused by viruses or bacteria. When the stools are cultured in the lab, bacteria such as salmonella, campylobacter or shigella may be found. Although infectious diarrhoea normally settles within three to four days, some cases may persist longer, and it is always important to check that no infection is present.

Many young persons developing persistent diarrhoea and abdominal pain suffer from irritable bowel syndrome (IBS). Here, there is no inflammation of the gut, and it appears to be completely normal on X-ray and at endoscopy. Various factors, such as chemicals produced by gut bacteria, or stress, lead to painful spasms in the muscles of the bowel wall, wind and diarrhoea.

In contrast to IBD, however, it is very unusual in patients with IBS to have diarrhoea during the night – it generally starts first thing in the morning. It's very important to tell your doctor if you are getting diarrhoea during the night (between 10 p.m. to 4 a.m.), as this usually means there is definite disease present somewhere in the bowel which must be fully investigated.

Doctors always check out common diseases before looking for those that are rarer, and so many young people with IBD are first labelled as having IBS. It's important, therefore, that blood tests to exclude IBD are done in all cases of suspected IBS.

Another fairly common cause of diarrhoea in young people is coeliac disease. Coeliac disease is an immune reaction to gluten – the main protein found in wheat, rye and barley. This reaction causes damage to the lining of the small intestine so that nutrients are not fully absorbed and pass out of the body, leading to diarrhoea and weight loss. A straightforward blood test (tissue transglutaminase) is available for screening for coeliac disease, and if this is positive, the diagnosis is confirmed by an endoscopic biopsy from the duodenum.

Diarrhoea sometimes accompanied by blood in the stool is a feature of certain sexually transmitted diseases and also of cancer of the colon. Colon cancer is very unusual in young people unless it runs in their families, but in people over the age of 45 with persistent diarrhoea with or without bleeding, X-ray or endoscopy must always be performed to ensure that there is no cancer present.

Diarrhoea may also be caused by diseases of organs outside the gut, such as the thyroid or the adrenal glands.

ABDOMINAL PAIN

Abdominal pain is a common feature of IBD, but again may arise from many other causes. It may arise not only in the gut but also in other abdominal organs, such as the kidneys, bladder, female reproductive organs or even when there are problems with the muscles of the abdominal wall. Because the nerve supply of the abdominal organs is not as precisely localised as that of other parts of the body, such as the hands or legs, the position of the pain may not be an accurate guide to the organ which is causing the trouble.

As a general rule, pains arising from organs in the first part of the gut, such as the stomach, duodenum and gall-bladder, are felt in the centre of the upper abdomen and those in the middle parts, such as the small intestine, are felt around the navel. Pains caused by disease of the large intestine are felt in the central lower abdomen just above the groin.

So when describing abdominal pain it's important not only to indicate the position of the pain, but also any factors that may relieve it or make it worse. Pain in IBD characteristically is worse after eating, which stimulates muscular activity (peristalsis) in the bowel and is relieved by passing a stool or wind, both of which reduce the pressure inside the large intestine.

Tell the doctor how severe the pain is. All pains are unpleasant, but some pains are more unpleasant than others! A simple guide is to describe the pain as:

Mild: you can carry on with whatever you are doing even though there is discomfort.

Moderate: it's difficult for you to carry on, and you need to look for some way of finding relief.

Severe: the pain is so bad that you have no choice but to stop whatever you are doing, and to go home and rest until it settles.

It is also important to note the pattern of the pain – at what time during the day it comes on, whether it is associated with other symptoms such as wind or abdominal bloating, and whether there is any long-term pattern, such as variation with different stages of the menstrual cycle in young women.

The more accurate the description of the pain that you provide, the more help it will be to your doctor in sorting out its cause.

WIND AND BLOATING

Another topic that may make your toes curl! Don't worry about the terminology. If you want to call a fart a fart, then call it a fart. Your doctor will appreciate your clarity. If such words stick on the tongue, then you could try 'rectal flatus' or 'rectal flatulence'. It's important to make it clear that the gas is coming from the bottom end, because wind from the top end (a burp or a belch for real precision) has a different significance. This wind is usually caused by swallowing air (or sometimes by disease in the gallbladder) and is a result of stress and anxiety.

Wind from the tail end, however, may be due to abnormal bacterial fermentation in the large intestine. It by no means always signifies serious disease but is often increased in IBD, and may smell foul.

How do you know you pass more wind than others? We all (even film stars and aristocrats) pass wind and it's difficult to judge the amount. Scientists tell us that the normal range is 8–13 farts a day! If you exceed this it may be very distressing, especially socially, but don't bother counting – what is more important is whether the wind causes bloating and discomfort. Sometimes the wind seems to get trapped and can be very uncomfortable. If this means you have to undo your skirt or jeans to relieve the pressure, tell your doctor. It will help to focus his thoughts on your offending large intestine. The wind in IBD is often more offensive (it contains more hydrogen sulphide) and if so you should mention it.

RECTAL BLEEDING

Bleeding from the anus is always worrying to patients as it can be a sign of cancer. However, by far the commonest cause is piles – swollen blood vessels around the anus that may bleed when hard pieces of stool pass through.

Rectal bleeding in IBD usually indicates inflammation in the lower large intestine.

In describing rectal bleeding to your doctor it is important that you tell him the following points:

- Is the blood bright (as when you cut yourself) or dark? Darkness suggests that it is old blood that has been shed higher up the intestine.

- Does it coat the stool or is it mixed in with it? If it coats the stool it is likely to be coming from, or very close to, the anus.

- Does it appear on the loo paper and drip into the lavatory pan? This is usually a clear sign of bleeding from piles.

- Melaena, that is, stools that are pitch-black, like tar, are a sign of bleeding high in the gut, usually from the stomach or duodenum. Bleeding from the caecum may not alter the stool colour at all, even though it is severe enough to lead to anaemia.

WEIGHT LOSS

Weight loss is caused by a range of diseases apart from IBD that are too numerous to mention here. However, it's an important symptom that should always put a doctor on the alert.

Weight loss is a common symptom in IBD and before seeing your doctor you should try and think whether or not you had any weight loss since your illness began. If you have not weighed yourself recently have you noticed any change in the fit of your clothes? Do you need to tighten your belt by a further notch?

OTHER IMPORTANT SYMPTOMS

A number of other less frequent symptoms may be caused by IBD. They may provide valuable pointers to the diagnosis so if you have suffered any of these problems, do not forget to tell your doctor about them.

Fatigue: this is a common problem in IBD. It may be the result of anaemia, sleeplessness from diarrhoea at night or simply the presence of a chronic inflammatory disease. However, fatigue also occurs in many other diseases ranging from thyroid problems to depression and always deserves careful investigation.

Fever: occurs in cases of IBD where there is very active inflammation. Again, it's a non-specific symptom occurring in many other conditions, but which should always lead to careful investigation.

Mouth ulcers: we are all familiar with painful white or yellow ulcers in our mouths and on our tongues. These are called 'aphthous' ulcers and they are usually of little importance. However, if they keep coming back very frequently and painfully it may be a pointer to IBD. Sometimes CD attacks the lining of the mouth itself and the ulcers are bigger, more persistent and painful.

Pain in the anus: pain in and around the anus occurs quite often in IBD. If it is associated with a red and tender swelling, an abscess is usually the cause. This may occur because of a 'fistula-in-ano' (see page 154), which is a well-known feature of CD, but may occur quite independently. Pain in passing a stool, sometimes with bleeding as well, may mean a split in the lining of the anus, called a 'fissure-in-ano'.

Vaginal discharge: an offensive or discoloured vaginal discharge may indicate the presence of a fistula developing between the rectum and the vagina.

Red and inflamed eyes: IBD may lead to symptoms in organs beyond the gastrointestinal tract. The eyes are sometimes affected. Red gritty eyes may be a sign of episcleritis. Sometimes the inflammation is more severe, when the condition is known as uveitis. Eye symptoms must always be investigated promptly.

Joint pain and swelling: this is common in IBD and in some studies has affected 30% of patients. Low backache may be produced by inflammation of the joints between the lower part of the back bone known as the sacrum and the ilium, which is the upper part of the pelvis. This is known as 'sacroiliitis' and can be diagnosed on X-rays. Arthritis may also arise in other joints, particularly the ankles, knees, wrists and elbows.

Skin lesions: when IBD is very active, tender purplish red nodules may appear on the skin particularly on the shins.

These are called *erythema nodosum* and usually disappear when the IBD is brought under control. A less common skin problem is pyoderma gangrenosum. Pus-filled blisters appear on the skin often of the legs and they break down to form a deep red ulcer, which can be very difficult to heal.

Swollen and painful legs: because an inflammatory reaction may lead to an increase in the number of platelets in the blood, there is sometimes an increased risk of blood clots forming in IBD. A clot in the leg is known as a deep vein thrombosis (DVT) and may cause pain, swelling, coolness, aching and tenderness in the legs. Sometimes a clot in the leg vein may break off and travel to the lung causing a dangerous blockage to the circulation – a pulmonary embolus. This causes faintness, chest pain and breathlessness. It is a medical emergency, but fortunately uncommon in IBD, except after surgery when your surgical team will give you treatment to prevent it.

SYMPTOM SCORES

Sometimes doctors use symptom scores to assess a patient's response to treatment. The Harvey and Bradshaw index, for example, is used in Crohn's disease. The patient's general well-being, pain severity, stool frequency and disease complications, together with the presence of any abdominal masses, are all added together to give a number that provides a general idea of just how much better the disease may be. A number of such symptom scores exists. The Walmsley index, for example, is used in UC. There is no need at all for you to worry about them – but they may be the reason why your doctor always seems to be asking the same questions!

CHAPTER 4

Investigation of IBD

The investigation of IBD should not be a matter of chance or inspired guesswork, but a methodical process leading to understanding the damage that has been caused to the gut and the best way to repair it or to relieve its effects.

There are five stages:

1. Confirmation of the presence of IBD
2. Determination of its extent and activity
3. Identification of which type of IBD is present
4. Search for any complications
5. Selection of appropriate treatment

1. CONFIRMATION OF THE PRESENCE OF IBD

The most important investigations to confirm or exclude IBD are:

HISTORY AND EXAMINATION

This is the single most important step in sorting out your problems. After taking a detailed account of your symptoms and questioning you about them, your doctor will have a pretty good idea of what is going on, and the various investigations that may be ordered are usually done for confirmation rather than in the hope of throwing up new possibilities. It is vital therefore that you give a full account of what you have been experiencing and answer the doctor's questions as clearly as possible.

Do not be embarrassed! None of us likes to discuss the way our bowels are behaving or the appearance of our stools, but you must remember that your doctor has taken similar histories from many other patients before you and will take it in his or her stride. Do not try to use terms like 'tummy trouble' or 'bowel upset'. These are far too vague. The doctor needs to know exactly what is happening.

Many people are not sure which words to use to describe changes in their bowel functions. The medical terms for solid excrement is 'faeces', but simple words like 'poo' or 'number two' are perfectly acceptable. 'Stools' is a neutral term that is favoured by many. Likewise, you can talk about wind as 'flatus' or flatulence. Stools can easily be described as 'firm', 'soft', 'runny' (like soup), or 'watery' when they are completely liquid.

Before your appointment with the doctor try to think about what you want to say and get your story clear in your mind. Think about factors that may affect any pains you have had, as described in the last chapter. If you like, write it down so you don't forget anything you believe is important. If you are really embarrassed you could write some of your most worrying symptoms down on a piece of paper so that the doctor can read it, rather than having to describe them yourself.

When the story of the illness is clear, the doctor will ask further questions to widen his knowledge of factors which may be affecting your health, to check for complications and to find out about your previous health, your family and your social habits.

Usually the doctor will perform a physical examination immediately after taking the history. You will be asked to undress and the doctor will feel your abdomen for tenderness and any unusual lumps or bumps. It may be necessary to check your heart, lungs and limbs. If an examination of the rectum is required, the doctor will put on a rubber glove and lubricate it so that a finger will pass easily into the rectum. Although this may sound alarming, it is not usually painful. However, never forget that a doctor cannot perform any examination or test without your consent! If you would like a chaperone, just ask for one.

SIGMOIDOSCOPY

If IBD is suspected the doctor will often go straight on to do a sigmoidoscopy. You will be asked to lie on your left side with your knees drawn up and your bottom on the very edge of the couch. After passing a finger into the rectum to allow the muscles around the anus to relax, the doctor will introduce a slim, well-lubricated plastic tube (not much bigger than the finger) into the rectum. This has a light inside to enable the doctor to see up the bowel. Some air will be pumped in to distend the bowel allowing a better view. The sigmoidoscope will then slowly be advanced up the bowel as far as is comfortable – usually about 20cm. This should not be at all painful. The doctor can immediately see if the bowel lining is inflamed and if it is this may provide immediate confirmation of the diagnosis of IBD. A small piece of tissue can be taken for examination under the microscope in the laboratory. This is called a biopsy and is quite painless; you will merely feel a slight tugging. There is a very slight risk of bleeding after a biopsy is taken so you may be asked to rest for a short time before leaving the clinic. When the examination is complete, the doctor removes the sigmoidoscope and you will be provided with some tissues to clear away the lubricant before getting dressed again.

If you have any pain in the abdomen, anus or any bleeding following a sigmoidoscopy, let your doctor know straight away.

BLOOD TESTS

These are often taken at the same time straight after the initial history and examination. Sometimes it may be necessary to attend for blood tests at a separate laboratory. Your doctor will decide which tests are necessary, but the ones commonly requested for cases of IBD are listed in the table below:

Full Blood Count (FBC)	This examines the various cells that circulate in the blood. It will pick up anaemia, which is common in cases of IBD where there has been bleeding from the bowel. An increase in white cells may occur with infection (e.g. an abscess or inflammation). The platelet count is often useful as an index of increased activity of inflammation in IBD and may be significantly raised in severe cases.
Kidney function test	This will demonstrate any dehydration or loss of sodium or potassium from the body in cases of diarrhoea.
Liver function test	This includes the level in the blood of a protein called albumin, which is secreted into the bowel from inflamed areas of the intestine. A low level suggests continuing disease activity. Complications of IBD such as gallstones or sclerosing cholangitis will lead to abnormal liver function test and sometimes even jaundice.

C-reactive protein (CRP)	This is a very valuable test in establishing IBD. This protein is raised in many infections and inflammatory conditions but a raised CRP in patients with diarrhoea and abdominal pain is highly suggestive of IBD. It is also very useful in following the effectiveness of treatment – the aim being to keep the level within normal limits.
Erythrocyte sedimentation rate (ESR)	Changes in the amount of protein such as albumin and CRP lead to alterations in the viscosity of the blood plasma and this in turn means that the red cells in a column of blood settle more quickly than usual. Thus the ESR is another useful indicator of the presence of inflammation in the body but may be affected by many other conditions as well.
Tissue transglutaminase	This enzyme is raised in patients with coeliac disease (see page 48), which may coexist with IBD. It is therefore often determined during the investigation of patients suspected of having CD or colitis.
Thyroid-stimulating hormone (TSH)	As an overactive thyroid gland is a common cause of diarrhoea and weight loss, this test is often performed to ensure thyrotoxicosis has not been overlooked, but it has no direct effect on IBD or its treatment.

STOOL TESTS

Since infection is often a cause of diarrhoea, your doctor may want to send a stool sample to the laboratory to check for bacteria and parasites. You will be given a small plastic container with a spoon-shaped rod attached to the inside of the lid. When you have passed the stool, unscrew the lid and use the spoon to pick up a small amount of faeces about the size of a fingernail. Pop it in the top, screw it up tightly and deliver it back to your clinic as soon as possible. Don't forget to write your name and date of birth and any other details required on the label!

Faecal calprotectin

A stool test that may soon be widely used in order to establish IBD measures faecal calprotectin.

Calprotectin is a protein that is found in white blood cells. There is more calprotectin in a white cell than there is haemoglobin in a red cell, so you can see that it is a very important substance. It's particularly useful because it is a very stable compound. Calprotectin does not start to break down until it has been left on the bench at room temperature for a whole week! This stability makes it very useful in the management of IBD.

We have seen how IBD is caused by the body's immune system attacking the bacteria that live in the bowel. When this immune attack starts, white cells migrate from the blood through the lining of the bowel into the lumen. They are swept out of the body along with the faeces.

Normal faeces contain few if any white cells. In IBD many are present. In the old days we used to examine faeces for white cells under the microscope, but that was unpleasant. Nowadays it's possible to check for the presence of white cells in the faeces even when the sample is two to three days old by measuring the concentration of calprotectin present. If the calprotectin is raised, we know that more white cells are entering the faeces than is normal. This can occur in cases of cancer or infection, but if those have been excluded a raised concentration of faecal calprotectin is strongly suggestive of IBD. Indeed, in some hospitals it is used as a screening test to differentiate patients with IBS, where little inflammation is present, from true cases of IBD.

Up to now calprotectin tests have not been widely available and have mainly been used on a research basis. As we become more aware of the value of this test, however, it will become available more easily. Apart from distinguishing cases of IBD from other forms of diarrhoea, I have found it particularly useful in assessing the response of patients to treatment. When IBD is switched off whether by diet or drugs, the faecal calprotectin falls back to normal levels. This may be particularly useful in deciding how long to keep patients with resistant CD on enteral feeding. I once had a patient who was very keen to control his CD by diet, but kept having early relapses and had failed to establish a long-term diet on which he could remain well. We started him again on elemental diet and checked his faecal calprotectin at weekly intervals. We found that it took a full nine weeks for his calprotectin to come down to normal levels. Fortunately he was willing to continue with enteral feeding for such a long period of time. Such a long course of treatment is not usually necessary but in this instance it proved to be highly beneficial as the patient was then able to reintroduce normal food items and to build up his individual diet in the usual way without the setbacks he had previously been suffering. He successfully entered long-term remission.

Faecal calprotectin is also helpful in deciding how severe a case of IBD may be. Clearly those cases with very high levels are more severe than those where the calprotectin is barely raised at all and this may influence the doctor's choice of treatment – for example, very high levels in CD might indicate the need for treatment with an initial course of corticosteroids as well as elemental diet. Occasional calprotectin testing on patients reintroducing foods will be a very useful way of confirming that the diets they establish are indeed the correct ones to keep their conditions well under control.

2. DETERMINATION OF DISEASE EXTENT AND ACTIVITY

If the first round of investigations confirms that the patient's symptoms are likely to be caused by IBD, stage 2 determines where in the gut the inflammation is and its severity.

To do this we need to get some kind of picture of the gastrointestinal tract. This may be done by radionuclide scanning, X-rays or endoscopy.

The determination of the extent of the disease is important as this may give valuable clues as to the type of IBD that is present and also may affect treatment. Evidence of inflammation in the small bowel strongly supports a diagnosis of CD, but if the changes appear to be old rather than new and are in the lower part of the ileum, then it may be that symptoms are caused by bile-salt spill over, rather than acute inflammation, and the treatment will differ.

There are three main ways of getting this picture of the bowel:

1. **Scans with radioisotope** – the leucocyte or white cell scan is a very valuable investigation for confirming the presence of IBD and assessing its extent and severity. White cells are separated from the blood and labelled

with a very small amount of radioactive material (indium or technetium). The white cells are then injected back into the bloodstream and as they are still alive, will go about their usual tasks. This means they go to areas such as the liver, spleen and the bone marrow where white cells are commonly stored. However, they also go to sites of active inflammation, including areas of IBD in the gut or an abscess anywhere in the body. Thus they may give a very clear picture of exactly where there is inflammation in the gut and its activity is reflected in the strength of the signal so that it's possible to see whether there is mild or severe damage. What's more, any abscesses that may be present can easily be seen.

In hospitals with a good department of nuclear medicine, white cell scanning is enormously valuable in managing cases of IBD. However, not all hospitals have access to nuclear medicine; sometimes patients have to be sent off to other centres. Under these circumstances the delay involved in waiting for the result may be too long for doctors and patients wanting to get ahead with treatment as fast as possible.

If you are sent for a white cell scan, there is no preparation prior to the test and you may eat and drink normally. The test is carried out in two phases. In phase 1 about 40mls of blood is taken from a vein in your arm and the white cells are separated from it by centrifuging. They are then labelled with a very small amount of radioactive chemical and re-injected back into the bloodstream. This part of the test can take up to two hours.

In phase 2, usually performed one to four hours later, the patient is scanned with a gamma camera producing a picture on which dark areas are seen as the site of inflammation. White cells may enter an abscess more slowly than they enter the gut and if an abscess is suspected, patients are sometimes recalled the following day for a further scan.

No particular after care is needed for white cell scanning. The great advantage of white cell scanning is that it displays the whole gut in one picture, which is not the case with other investigations.

2. **X-rays** – the simplest X-ray that may be helpful in IBD is a plain X-ray of the abdomen. This is a simple, quick and painless examination – just like having your photo taken. It does not require any special preparation and usually can be performed immediately after your clinic appointment. It is not particularly good at outlining all the bowel that is affected by IBD, but it may show the presence of right-sided (proximal) constipation in the presence of left-sided (distal) inflammatory bowel disease. It may also show dilatation of the colon, that is to say swelling caused by stricture formation or severe inflammation, as may be seen in toxic megacolon. Sometimes complications such as an abscess or perforation may be apparent on straight abdominal films. As the test is simple and quick, it is very often repeated in the course of treatment of patients with severe UC and in particular to get early warning of any of the serious complications mentioned above.

Barium enema: this involves barium sulphate – a liquid preparation that is opaque to X-rays and therefore shows up on X-ray films. It is used to investigate diseases of the large intestine. Sometimes the barium may flow back through the ileo-caecal valve into the lower small intestine and demonstrate inflammation there. A barium enema, therefore, is primarily used to assess UC. It shows the presence of inflammation very clearly but also can pick up strictures and dilatation. It may be dangerous to do a barium enema when the bowel is severely dilated as very occasionally perforations may occur in this situation. It is obviously of little value in investigating small bowel disease and does not pick up complications arising outside the bowel.

A barium enema involves considerable preparation, which may be a disadvantage. Prior to the test all faeces have to be cleared from the bowel by means of strong laxatives and a special diet; specific details will vary from one hospital to another. It's usual on the day of preparation to eat low-residue foods. This might involve a boiled egg with white toast for breakfast together with black tea or coffee. Lunch is based on white meat or fish with boiled or mashed potato or rice and no fruit or vegetables. Jelly, yoghurt, fruit squashes and again black tea or coffee are permissible. For supper, the evening before the X-ray, it's usual to avoid all solid food completely but clear soup (consommé), jelly, black tea and coffee and fruit squash are allowable.

During this day a powerful laxative, such as Picolax or Citromag, is given which will produce vigorous diarrhoea to empty the bowel; it is important to drink liberal amounts of fluid to prevent dehydration. You should drink a glass of water every hour. After midnight, however, patients are usually kept nil by mouth except for their usual medication, although if the X-ray appointment is in the afternoon, a light breakfast as mentioned above, is given.

On arriving in the X-ray department, the barium is administered through a tube inserted into the rectum. An injection of a drug called Buscopan is given to relax the bowel muscle as spasm may prevent the flow of barium round the colon. After the bowel has been filled, the barium is then allowed to drain out and a moderate amount of air is pumped in. This distends the gut and allows 'double contrast' images to be taken, in which the lining of the gut coated in barium stands out clearly against the radiolucent air inside the bowel itself. This enables the radiologist to see quite small lesions such as ulcers or polyps. In order to get better views during the examination, the radiologist will ask you to turn into various positions on the X-ray table which may also be tilted up or down.

After the test patients are encouraged to try and expel the remaining barium from the bowel. Sometimes a laxative solution may be given to help this. If too much barium is left inside, it may set and cause severe constipation. I well remember a most undignified half-hour which I spent digging cement-like barium out of the tail end of a most embarrassed patient. For two to three days after a barium enema, the bowel motions will be white due to persisting barium.

Barium meal and follow through: this is an examination of the small intestine. Barium can also be used to examine the stomach, although nowadays it's more usual to do a gastroscopy instead. The barium used to examine the stomach is thicker than that used to look at the small bowel and so it's uncommon for both stomach and small bowel to be examined on the same occasion. X-rays can be taken as the barium passes along the small intestine until it passes into the large intestine. The presence of faeces here does not usually spoil the images obtained, although some radiologists will prepare the bowel as for an enema so that it is empty and then pump air into the rectum as barium is passing from small bowel to large. This is called a pneumocolon and with a barium follow through these together may give very valuable information on the state of the lower small bowel and the caecum. A barium follow through therefore is of particular value in the assessment of CD.

Sometimes radiologists prefer to pass barium into the duodenum (the first part of the small bowel) through a special tube rather than just allowing the patient to drink the barium. This is because the rate of passage of barium from the stomach into the intestine can then be controlled more precisely. A barium X-ray done this way is called an enteroclysis.

For straightforward barium follow through there is no special preparation. The patient is asked not to eat or drink for six hours prior to the examination and normal medications may be taken. On arrival in the X-ray department a barium drink is given and the radiologist takes a series of images as the barium passes along the small intestine. The patient is again often asked to change position in order to get a better image. Graded compression to the abdomen is often applied in order to separate overlapping bowel loops. The speed at which the barium passes along the small bowel varies from less than an hour to more than four hours and it may be necessary to wait in the department for some time while the barium passes on and a series of films is obtained.

After the examination the stools will again be white for a few days as the barium passes through and some departments recommend a mild laxative to prevent the barium leading to constipation. The patient is able to eat and drink normally after the examination.

CT – scan and virtual colonoscopy: in CT scanning a series of X-rays of the body are taken from different angles and are coordinated by the computer into images which look like slices through the body at various levels. CT scans have been one of the most dramatic improvements in our investigation of the gastrointestinal tract in recent years and have made exploratory abdominal surgery (the old laparotomy) largely a thing of the past. Even more recent computer advances have allowed the reconstruction from these X-ray series, of a view of the large bowel which is in many ways as good as that given by an endoscope. This is known as CT colonography or virtual colonoscopy. It also has the benefit that the bowel examination is not limited by the presence of strictures or tumours that might prevent the onward passage of an endoscope. CT scanning and virtual colonoscopy have therefore become very popular, particularly in investigating the colon in the elderly or those who are frail, as in order to get the best pictures it is the position of the X-ray machinery that moves rather than the patient. Furthermore, contrast medium can be given to clarify differences between different tissues, and the CT scan has the further advantage of allowing pictures of abdominal organs which are outside the gut and therefore not visible on barium X-rays or at endoscopy.

As experience increases, some radiologists may come to prefer CT to barium enemas in the assessment of cases of UC, but CT scanning is less good at picking up lesions in the small bowel.

If you are sent for a CT scan to examine the large intestine, preparation will be as for barium enema. On the day of the examination you should not eat or drink for six hours before the examination.

You will be asked to lie down on the X-ray table and a tube will be inserted into your rectum. CO_2 is used to inflate your colon through this tube. Various contrast media and Buscopan, a drug to relieve abdominal pain, may be injected through a cannula placed in a vein on the back of your hand or wrist. When the examination starts you will hear various noises as the X-ray machine moves around. Images are taken with you lying on your back and then on your front. When the examination is over you are able to eat and drink normally and no particular precautions need to be taken.

Magnetic Resonance Imaging (MRI): MRI differs from CT scanning in that no X-rays are involved. It relies on the use of a strong magnetic field to align the nuclear magnetisation of the hydrogen atoms in water which, when altered by different radio frequency fields, emit a signal. This signal is detected by the scanner and reformatted into multiple images of the body. It provides much more powerful soft tissue resolution than CT and is particularly useful in assessing diseases of the brain, muscles and circulatory system as well as in cancer imaging.

MRI is particularly useful in imaging the small bowel. It is customary to get the patient to drink some water first as this contains many hydrogen ions and will fill the bowel satisfactorily. An intravenous contrast agent is often administered. A series of pictures can then be taken which are usually as good as those obtained from barium follow throughs, but MRI has the great advantage that repeated examinations can be performed without the anxiety of excess exposure to radiation.

The main disadvantage of MRI is that some patients feel claustrophobic when lying in the instrument.

3. **Endoscopy** – some people get rather confused about endoscopy because there appear to be so many different words which end in the same way. Thus there may be gastroscopy, colonoscopy, bronchoscopy and cystoscopy as well as several others. In fact it's all very simple. The suffix -scopy means looking and endo- means

inside, thus endoscopy just means looking inside and can be applied to an examination anywhere in the body. If we are being specific about which organ is being studied, then we change the prefix endo- to something representing the organ in question. Therefore gastro- implies examination of the stomach, colono- examination of the bowel, broncho- examination of the airways or bronchial tubes and cysto-examination of the bladder. The most important forms of endoscopy for IBD are colonoscopy, enteroscopy and gastroscopy.

Colonoscopy: this is an examination of the large bowel or colon by means of a flexible instrument that is passed through the anus. The instrument has a video camera at one end and the image is transmitted to a TV screen on which the doctor gets good views of the lining of the bowel. Apart from the video connections the endoscope can also suck out excess fluid or waste in the bowel and pump air in, so that the bowel can be distended in order to be seen more clearly. It's also possible to pass instruments down the channel to the end of the instrument. These can be used to take biopsies or to remove polyps or other lesions which the endoscopist may encounter.

Endoscopy has the advantage over X-rays that if something abnormal is seen, biopsies can be taken for examination in the laboratory to demonstrate their exact nature. Furthermore, instruments can be passed all the way along the large bowel and into the lower part of the small bowel, thus giving a good idea of the extent of the disease. Inflammation and ulcers can be clearly seen and the shape and size of these may be of value when deciding whether CD or UC is present. The disadvantages of colonoscopy are that it tends to be rather more uncomfortable than X-rays, so it's usual to sedate patients for the examination. There is also a very small risk (1 in 1,000) of making a hole in the bowel wall (perforation) or causing bleeding. These risks particularly arise when polyps are being removed.

Preparation for a colonoscopy begins on the previous day when a strong laxative (Picolax or Citromag) is given in order to clear the bowel of faeces so that good views of the mucosa may be seen. As with a barium enema it is customary to advise a low-residue diet beforehand and to emphasise the need to drink a glass of water every hour until the effect of the laxatives has worn off.

Patients should not eat for at least six hours before the examination. On arrival in the endoscopy department, the patient is asked to put on a hospital gown and to sign a form giving informed consent to the procedure. The examination takes place on a couch in theatre with a nurse assisting throughout to support and guide the patient. The doctor places a small cannula in the back of the hand or wrist and through this injects some sedation to make the patient sleepy and relaxed. He then passes the instrument through the anus and along the bowel, inflating the bowel with some air as he proceeds in order to get better views and sucking out any excess fluid that may remain. As the instrument passes round tight bends in the bowel, there may be a little discomfort and the increased pressure in the bowel may make patients feel that they need to pass a motion, but this is, of course, most unlikely to happen as the bowel has already been emptied.

The examination can take anything from 20 minutes to an hour and it may be necessary to change position from time to time in order to help progress of the endoscope around to the caecum.

Once the caecum or terminal ileum is reached, the endoscope is slowly withdrawn. The doctor takes biopsies as necessary on the way out and may remove any polyps that he sees for examination in laboratory.

Following removal of the instrument, the patient is left to relax and recover. There is often a feeling of bloating because of the wind that has been instilled into the bowel but the endoscopist tries to remove as much of this air as possible before the examination is completed and any bloating usually settles quickly. Once the sedation has worn off the doctor sees the patient and explains his findings. It's a good idea to have someone with you at this time because a person who has been sedated frequently forgets things that may be important.

After the examination the sedation continues to circulate through the system and you should spend your time very quietly. In particular, you must not drive for 24 hours afterwards so you will certainly need an escort home after the colonoscopy. During the following 24 hours you should not operate any dangerous machinery, make any important decisions and should not drink alcohol, which may have a more intoxicating effect when taken on top of the sedation.

A small amount of bleeding may occur following the procedure because of bleeding from biopsy sites. However, if this continues or increases you should inform your doctor without delay. Likewise, slight discomfort from residual air after the examination in the bowel should clear quite quickly. Immediately inform your doctor if there is persisting or increasing pain.

It is customary to go back to the clinic a few days after the colonoscopy in order to discuss the results of the biopsies, which, of course, take a little while to be processed in the laboratory.

Flexible sigmoidoscopy: sometimes when it is believed that the disease is limited to the left side of the colon, it may be sufficient to perform a flexible sigmoidoscopy rather than a full colonoscopy. In this, the endoscope is passed through the anus in the same way, but the instrument is only advanced as far as the splenic flexure, that is to say only the left side of the bowel is examined. Because of this, the preparation does not need to be as thorough. Usually patients are given a small enema just before the examination to enable the left side to be cleared of faeces. Because this is the simpler examination, it may sometimes be performed without sedation.

As with colonoscopy the advantages are that the lining of the bowel can be seen very clearly and biopsies can be taken, strictures dilated and polyps removed.

The risks and after-effects are the same as those described for colonoscopy, but as the examination is much shorter and quicker, the risk of complication is much less.

Enteroscopy: an endoscopic examination of the small intestine. This needs a much slimmer instrument than used for colonoscopy as, of course, the small bowel is smaller than the large! For many years it was not very popular amongst doctors because the length of the small intestine made it very difficult to get an instrument all the way along it. However, a recent development in Japan called double-balloon enteroscopy has made this technique much more practicable. In this technique there is a balloon at the end of the enteroscope and there is also a transparent over-tube through which the enteroscope can slide easily. This over-tube also has a balloon.

Double-balloon enteroscopy can be done either from

above passing the instrument through the mouth, or from below passing it through the rectum and up into the terminal ileum. Once the instrument is in the small bowel, the balloon at the end of the enteroscope is blown up so that it presses firmly against the bowel wall. The enteroscope is then pulled back until the tip comes to lie at the mouth of the over-tube. At this stage the balloon on the over-tube is inflated to hold the small bowel in place. The balloon at the tip of the enteroscope is let down so that the tip can then pass further along the small bowel examining another section, which in turn will be pulled back to the over-tube to be held in place by the second balloon there. In this way the whole of the small bowel may be examined. Biopsies may be taken, polyps removed and strictures can be dilated.

A key disadvantage of this double-balloon method is the time required to visualise the small bowel. This can be longer than three hours, thus the examination is usually done under general anaesthetic and may mean that patients have to be admitted to hospital. Furthermore, this technique is only available at a limited number of specialist centres.

Nevertheless, the use of double-balloon enteroscopy in the future may significantly improve our management of small bowel with strictures and mean that many patients that would previously have had to undergo surgery may now be treated endoscopically with complete success.

Gastroscopy: this type of endoscopic examination of the oesophagus, stomach and duodenum is sometimes abbreviated to OGD. It is not as important in IBD as other forms of endoscopy because UC never affects the upper gut and although there may be occasional cases of CD damaging the oesophagus or causing inflammation in the stomach and duodenum, these are quite unusual.

It's a much simpler examination than a colonoscopy. The only preparation required is for the patient to fast for six hours beforehand so that the stomach is empty.

On arrival at the endoscopy department, the patient is often offered a choice between having sedation in the same way as for colonoscopy, or merely to have the back of the throat anaesthetised with a spray. The advantage of the latter is that the patient recovers very quickly and there are no problems about driving or using dangerous machinery in the next 24 hours.

If sedation is chosen a vein on the back of the hand or wrist is cannulated and sedation administered in exactly the same way as for colonoscopy. If local anaesthetic is chosen, the doctor will spray the back of the throat with liquid, often tasting of bananas, which acts very quickly. The patient then lies on their left side. A mouth guard is inserted to prevent any damage to the patient's teeth or to the endoscope itself.

The endoscopist then passes the slim instrument into the back of the throat, down the oesophagus and into the stomach, which is distended with air to enable better views to be obtained. The endoscopist may examine the duodenum.

As with other forms of endoscopy, biopsies can be taken and polyps removed. The examination is usually quite quick, taking only a few minutes, after which the endoscope is removed and the patient allowed to recover. There are rarely any after-effects. The patient may belch a little of the air which has been used to distend the stomach, but it is unusual to get any pain or discomfort.

3. IDENTIFICATION OF WHICH TYPE OF IBD IS PRESENT

Once the extent of inflammation through the bowel is known, the doctors may have a very good idea as to which sort of IBD is present. A left-sided colitis is nearly always UC. Extensive disease in the small bowel can confidently be diagnosed as CD.

Nevertheless, to make a complete diagnosis, it is always a good idea to have biopsies.

Biopsies are small pieces of tissue only a few millimetres across which are obtained at endoscopy from affected parts of the gut. It's customary to take them from not only parts of the gut that are inflamed but also from adjoining areas that are not. Sometimes microscopic changes may indicate that the extent of the disease is greater than was thought from X-rays and endoscopy alone and changes may be seen under the microscope that cast valuable light on the type of IBD present. As an example granulomas present in biopsies from the large intestine may strongly support a diagnosis of CD, even though there is no small bowel involvement.

The main differences between UC and CD are summarised in the table on page 17. It is important to remember that although inflammation may be present in the large intestine, its pattern under the microscope may not be typical of either CD or UC. Often, the pathologist is unable to make a definite diagnosis. This does not inevitably mean that a diagnosis of an indeterminate colitis may be reached. Other factors, such as the pattern of distribution of inflammation, may push the diagnosis one way or another. For this reason, the pathologist may well say that the changes seen under the microscope are 'consistent' with CD or UC, even though they are not fully diagnostic. This does not mean that he has made a definite diagnosis, but merely that the changes would be in line with such a diagnosis if other features of the case support it. This is an important distinction to make as it sometimes leads to patients being labelled with the wrong form of IBD and therefore being given less than ideal treatment.

4. SEARCH FOR ANY COMPLICATIONS

Your doctor will now have a good idea of what is going on in your gut. He may need, however, further information as to whether any particular complication has arisen and to do this he may order some of the following tests:

Bone density: some patients with IBD have thinning of the bones. An early degree of bone thinning is called osteopaenia. More severe damage is called osteoporosis. This may lead to increased fragility as thin bones fracture more easily after relatively minor trauma or the bodies of the vertebrae become crushed. Fortunately, nowadays treatment is available to correct these problems.

Bone thinning of this sort may be caused by the inflammation of IBD itself, or by a diet poor in calcium and vitamin D. Most commonly it is due to long-term treatment with corticosteroids.

Osteoporosis and osteopaenia can be detected by a bone-density determination. This is an X-ray examination performed to measure the thickness of bones in the body, usually in the hip and spine. The amount of radiation used is small, but nevertheless it should not be carried out during pregnancy.

As a preparation, all metal objects must be removed from the area to be scanned as these may deflect X-rays. You will be asked to lie on your back on the X-ray couch. When spinal X-rays are performed the legs are raised on a cushion. You must remain still during the procedure but may talk freely. The arm of the X-ray machine is then passed over the area several times and pictures taken.

After the test the scans are reviewed and the bone density determined and compared to the normal range of someone of your age. The results are sent to your doctor for the next clinic appointment.

Hydrogen breath test: hydrogen is a gas that is present in the atmosphere in minute amounts. It's also produced in the human body by the fermentation of carbohydrate in the diet by the bacteria that live in the bowel. Normally, such bacteria are found only in the large intestine, but when the bowel is damaged by Crohn's disease, the small bowel may also be colonised and this may cause unpleasant symptoms including wind, pain and diarrhoea. Hydrogen produced in the bowel is absorbed into the bloodstream, taken to the lungs and excreted on the breath.

Therefore, a hydrogen breath test can show if there are bacteria growing in the small intestine. It's also useful to check for malabsorption of certain sugars, which may be digested with difficulty, such as the milk sugar lactose or the fruit sugar fructose.

It's necessary to have an overnight fast before the test and as gases produced by cigarette smoke may interfere with the measurement; there should be no smoking from 6 p.m. the previous day.

The test itself is simple and painless and takes about three and a half hours. Samples of the breath are taken by breathing through a special mouthpiece from which samples of expired air can be sucked into a syringe. The gas in the syringe is then injected into a hydrogen measuring machine and the result is quickly available.

It's normal to take a sample on arrival in the department as the base line. After this you will be asked to drink a standard amount of a sugar solution. The type of sugar that is used will depend on what your doctor is looking for. If he is looking for bacterial overgrowth, for instance, it's customary to use glucose. Samples of breath are then taken in just the same way in half-hourly intervals.

If the level of hydrogen on the breath is more than 20 parts per million, in the fasting sample, or if it rises above that level after drinking the sugar solution, it shows that the sugar is reaching the bacteria somewhere in the gut and the test is positive. Subsequent action depends on what the doctor is looking for; if he finds that there is bacterial overgrowth he may recommend antibiotics to clear it or if he finds evidence of malabsorption of lactose, he may put you on a low-lactose diet.

Intestinal permeability test: this is a simple painless test to see if there is damage to the small intestine making it more permeable to large molecules, which should not, under normal circumstances, be able to pass through the intestinal wall. It may be of value in confirming inflammation in CD.

It is necessary to avoid alcohol for 48 hours before the test as this in itself can affect intestinal permeability. So may certain medications such as aspirin and other non-steroidal anti-inflammatory drugs (see page 40). These should not be taken for 24 hours before the test and you also should have fasted from midnight. Just before the test is started, two or three cups of clear fluids (water, fruit squash, black tea or coffee) should be taken to ensure that an adequate volume of urine will be passed.

A sweet test solution will be given to you to drink. This contains the sugars to be used that have been labelled with a small amount of radioactivity. The customary sugars are

^{51}Cr-EDTA and ^{14}C-mannitol; some departments may use other sugars.

After one hour from the start of the test you will be able to eat and drink normally, but no alcohol must be taken until it has been completed. For the next six hours all urine is collected into a container provided. At the end of six hours you should take care to empty the bladder to make sure that all urine passed during this period is contained in the collection. The completed container is returned to the department of nuclear medicine for measurement of the amounts of sugar which it contains.

Mannitol is normally absorbed completely and all this sugar should therefore be present in the urine. EDTA is a larger molecule and does not pass through the intestinal wall. It is therefore not absorbed into the bloodstream and should not be present in the urine. The damage that has occurred to the wall of the small intestine may be calculated by relating the amount of EDTA in the collected urine to the amount of mannitol.

Magnetic Resonance Imaging (MRI): we have discussed this earlier (page 69). The advent of MRI has been of enormous help in detecting certain complications of IBD, in particular the damage to the bile ducts which occurs in sclerosing cholangitis (page 162) and also in sorting out the anatomy of fistulae round the anus, which may be very complicated. The soft tissue images that an MRI provides are invaluable in looking at those particular problems.

SeHCAT: this is short for 75-selenium homotaurocholic acid retention test, but there is no need at all to remember such a long name! SeHCAT is merely a bile acid that has been labelled with some radioactive selenium so that it can easily be detected.

Bile acids are very important in digesting fat. As mentioned in chapter 1, because fat is not soluble in water, it is difficult to get fat-splitting enzymes into contact with it. Bile salts are the way the body gets round this problem. One end of each bile salt molecule is water soluble and the other fat soluble. In the gut they form little aggregates known as micelles. Fat enters these micelles and can be digested within them. They are thus very important in fat digestion.

Because they are so important, bile salts are recycled. They are produced in the liver and pass out in the bile when a fatty meal is eaten, and when the fat has been digested, they are reabsorbed so that they can go back in the blood to the liver and then be used over again. The part of the gut which does this reabsorption is in the terminal ileum at the very bottom of the small intestine. This part of the bowel is often damaged by CD and when this happens, the bile salts can no longer be reabsorbed. They therefore pass into the large intestine, which they irritate, causing diarrhoea. Patients with small bowel CD may therefore get diarrhoea which is due not to the inflammation to the bowel wall that the disease produces, but simply because bile salts are no longer reabsorbed.

The SeHCAT is designed to show whether bile salts can be reabsorbed or not. A small amount of the isotope is taken by mouth and after a short delay to allow its absorption you will be asked to enter a whole body scanner. This is a small cabin usually made of thick steel of the sort used in gun turrets in Second World War battleships! This is so thick that radioactivity from outside cannot penetrate it. Inside is a gamma camera that can measure the total radioactivity emitted by the patient.

After an initial reading has been taken you will be allowed to go home and asked to live normally for the following week, after which you will return to the department of nuclear medicine. Here you will once again be put into the whole body scanner and the total body radiation re-measured.

It's then possible to determine how much of the dose of radioactivity remains in the body. After seven days it's normal for more than 12% to be retained, but in patients with damage to the terminal ileum, there may be less than 5% still present. This then will provide the doctor with clear evidence whether the terminal ileum is absorbing bile salts adequately or not.

Serum vitamin B12 and red-cell folate: vitamin B12 and folic acid are both very important for the production of normal blood cells. Folic acid is found in green vegetables and vitamin B12 in meat and dairy products. They are both absorbed in the small intestine, folic acid in the jejunum and vitamin B12 in the ileum. Patients with small bowel Crohn's disease therefore may have a deficiency of these vitamins.

The amount of vitamin B12 and folic acid in the body can be determined by taking a blood sample from the arm. Folic acid content is measured in the red cells, and the vitamin B12 in the serum.

Ultrasound: ultrasonography is the production of images of internal organs by means of very high-pitched sound waves inaudible to the human ear. Once these sound waves hit organs they produce echoes, which are reflected back to the receiver and built up into an image on a screen by a computer. Ultrasound is quick, painless and relatively straightforward and it is of great value in the detection of disease in the gallbladder, liver, pancreas and kidney.

Before an abdominal ultrasound, you will be asked to have nothing to eat or drink for six hours. This helps to ensure that the gallbladder is full of bile. If the gallbladder itself is to be examined, the previous day's supper should be fat-free. You may take your normal medication.

If a pelvic ultrasound is being prepared, the bladder should be full and it is necessary to drink plenty of fluid an hour before the examination and not pass urine until after it is over.

While you are lying comfortably on the couch, the radiologist will put some jelly on to your abdomen and move the transducer (sound-wave transmitter) over it. He may ask you to change position slightly as he examines different organs. The whole examination takes up to half an hour. A pelvic ultrasound may also involve a separate vaginal examination in which a small probe is introduced into the vagina. This also transmits sound waves producing pictures on the screen. This probe is not painful, but may feel a little uncomfortable.

After the test you may eat and drink normally and the radiologist will send a report on the examination to your doctor.

X-ray of sacroiliac joints: patients with IBD often develop arthritis, and one of the commonest forms is inflammation of the joint between the lower part of the spine – the sacrum – and the upper rim of the pelvis – the ilium. Sometimes inflammation in the sacroiliac joint may extend into the spine itself, a condition known as ankylosing spondylitis, which may be associated with IBD.

Such inflammation may cause pain in the back and can easily be detected by a straightforward X-ray that requires no special preparation and is no more complex than having your photo taken.

As IBD may affect so many other parts of the body it is sometimes necessary to seek an opinion from other specialists. A woman with IBD, for example, who has a vaginal discharge may need gynaecological assessment to investigate the possibility of a fistula between the rectum and the vagina. Likewise, patients with red and sore eyes may need to see an ophthalmologist and if they have arthritis, a rheumatologist. The scope of the possible investigations ordered by other specialties such as these is beyond the range of the current book.

5. SELECTION OF TREATMENT

The information provided by these investigations should now give your doctor all he requires to offer you a logical treatment based on the current condition of IBD in your gut. Thus a patient presenting with pain and diarrhoea who has inflammation in the terminal ileum and in the caecum would be suitable for treatment to suppress inflammation either by drugs that reduce the activity of the immune system, such as prednisolone or infliximab, or by dietary treatment to reduce the bacterial stimulus which leads to the immune system attacking them. On the other hand, someone with previous CD who comes back with further diarrhoea after several years of disease and activity may have been shown to have a scarred and somewhat narrowed terminal ileum, but his symptoms are likely to be due to a spillover of bile salts rather than to acute inflammation. He would need to be treated with a resin to reabsorb the bile salts rather than by immunosuppressants or diet. The presence of osteoporosis would be a factor arguing against further use of corticosteroids. A low serum B12 level would be an indication for regular injections of the vitamin.

There is no room for guesswork. Every case of IBD needs individual assessment and logical treatment in the light of the pathology that has been demonstrated. There used to be a tendency, now fortunately passing, for doctors to think, as soon as the possibility of IBD was raised, that the patient should be on corticosteroids. You will see that this is far from correct. Treatment of each case may vary considerably and in order to get things right, we have to know what is going on.

CHAPTER 5

Diet and treatment of Crohn's disease

If you have been given a diagnosis of Crohn's disease you may be feeling rather disappointed. CD is a chronic disease, which although rarely fatal may, if not properly controlled, cause you considerable unhappiness and difficulty. However, the good news is that it can be successfully treated and that if you work together with your medical advisors to find the treatment that best suits you, there is no reason why you should not live a full and active life and achieve all the ambitions you have set yourself.

The first decision you must take, with the help of your doctor, is which way you would like to treat your CD.

As we have seen, CD is caused by an attack launched by the body's immune system on the bacteria that live in your bowel. It can therefore be treated by changing the bacteria's metabolisms so that they no longer attract the immune attack or it can be treated by suppressing the immune system so that the effects of the attack are eliminated.

The initial response of many patients is to say, 'Well, I have got a patch of inflamed intestine, why can't it be cut out?' The answer, of course, is that it can be.

Unfortunately, this rarely cures CD permanently: 90% of cases recur after surgery. Furthermore, removing part of the gut may lead to other complications, such as vitamin B12 deficiency, for example. It's true that if you perform a total colectomy and ileostomy, thereby taking away literally all the bacteria living in the bowel, the relapse rate is very much lower. Some authorities quote figures as low as 15%. Few patients, however, would like to start treatment by having an ileostomy and even then there is still the risk of recurrence in the small bowel. Often when complications occur, surgery is essential in CD and when followed up by careful medical treatment, the results can be very good indeed. However, most patients and most doctors would like to avoid surgery if they possibly can and usually put it low on their list of choices.

For many years gastroenterologists concentrated on immunosuppression to cope with CD. This still proves a very satisfactory treatment for many patients and is discussed in detail on page 117. Evidence is now accumulating, however, that changing the activity of the gut bacteria may be even more effective.

Immunosuppressive drugs do, of course, carry side-effects which are sometimes severe and suppressing the activity of the immune system carries its own dangers, not least of increasing the risk of infection and reactivation of TB. Furthermore, it's often relatively ineffective. Remission rates on corticosteroids are only about 60–70%. It's widely accepted that 50% of patients with CD will need to undergo surgery and these figures are taken from patients treated by immunosuppression.

Elemental diet is the most effective treatment currently available for CD because 80–90% of patients who are willing to continue with it for two to three weeks will go into remission. No other treatment can match these figures! In my opinion patients with proven CD would be very wise to give the diet method a trial.

If we are going to try to reduce the metabolic effects of gut bacteria therefore, the main choices available at present are antibiotics and diet.

ANTIBIOTICS

A number of antibiotics have been shown to be very valuable in the treatment of CD. These include metronidazole, ciprofloxacin and clarithromycin. Indeed, virtually any antibiotic that is effective against bacteria living in the gut may produce at least a temporary remission of CD.

In the short term, courses of antibiotics may be very helpful and may indeed enable you to avoid a course of prednisolone. In the long term, however, they usually are less than satisfactory. This is because antibiotics do not kill all the bacteria against which they are directed. In a case of pneumonia, for example, they may kill 70%, but the other 30% are mopped up by the body's white cells, which therefore have a much easier job than if antibiotics were not being used. There is a major difference in CD where there is no specific pathogen. The remaining bowel bacteria are not destroyed by white cells and when the antibiotics are stopped the 25–30% of bacteria remaining will rapidly grow back to the original level and trigger off the disease once more.

Furthermore, it's very common for bacteria to become resistant to antibiotics. Any attempt to control bacteria in the bowel requires regularly changing your antibiotic to a different preparation to try and avoid bacterial resistance. This becomes quite a tedious business and also risks the development of multi-resistant bacteria, which may pass from one person to another. This can lead to an increase in the number of strains of antibiotic-resistant bacteria spread through the population and this in turn makes treatment of infections caused by those bacteria all the more difficult.

Because of similarities between the appearances under the microscope and tuberculosis, several trials have been performed of the use of anti-tubercular antibiotics in CD.

Although these have been carried on for several months and have often involved the use of three or four anti-tubercular drugs together, they have not been shown to be effective.

This is not to say that antibiotics may not prove to have considerable value in years to come. There has already been some success in achieving remission by giving patients courses of suitable antibiotics together, and then following them up with a probiotic preparation such as VSL-#3. However, this type of treatment is still in its infancy and has yet to be proven in proper trials. Although it may sometimes be available in specialist IBD centres, it is not something to be used at an early stage in straight-forward cases.

NUTRITIONAL TREATMENT OF CD

Presently, therefore, the most reliable way of controlling bacterial activity is diet.

The basis of this treatment is that certain bacteria in the gut produce chemicals that trigger off the immune attack. These bacteria use undigested food residues coming down from the small intestine as their energy source. If they are deprived of these residues, their activity ceases and the disease settles. It is then possible to build up a diet of safe foods on which the patient remains well. The bacteria responsible for the trouble slowly die out, and after some years, the CD will have burnt itself out completely and the patient can go back to eating normally.

This works very well in the majority of our patients. However, there are challenges with diet. In the first place the diet is different from patient to patient. No one with CD starting on dietary therapy can know for certain what will suit him and what will not. Patients with coeliac disease are all given a gluten-free diet and 97% do very well indeed. One patient with CD, however, may be upset by wheat, another by maize and milk and yet another by chocolate and peanuts.

Although we know which foods are the most likely to cause trouble, there is so much individual variation that a long, slow process of food testing is necessary and this requires time and patience. It takes about three months for the patient to work out a diet accurately and during that time there will be one or two reactions as the foods are tested. During this period the patient must keep carefully to his diet. Admittedly, this is easier than, say, following a diet for weight loss, because the patient feels so very much better on a diet and is so pleased that his symptoms have settled. Nevertheless it takes considerable determination to keep to a diet over the months, particularly if this may mean avoiding a favourite food such as cake or biscuits. However, when the diet is followed correctly, the results are dramatic.

Furthermore, dietary therapy may not be available everywhere. Some hospitals do not have the specialist dietetic staff to be able to provide the support and reassurance that a patient may require. I hope that this book may help, in some way, to remedy that problem. If you want to try dietary treatment and your doctor says it is not possible, then perhaps your GP can refer you to a different hospital where the necessary staff are available.

The advantages of diet are that it gives the patient control over the disease. You decide what you eat and when you wish to be sure to be well, such as for an exam or wedding; the matter is in your own hands. If you keep to the diet you will remain in good health! What's more, diet has no side-effects and the risk of nasty complications, such as abscesses, is greatly reduced.

Finally, diet will often work where other treatments such as prednisolone and infliximab have failed. Because of these advantages, my own view is that everyone who has CD would be well advised to try dietary therapy because in the long term, the benefits are considerable.

ELEMENTAL DIET

Patients with CD frequently lose weight and become malnourished. It was the introduction of intravenous feeding – that is, feeding through a vein rather than by mouth to combat malnutrition – that led to the discovery of dietary treatment. Patients who required surgery were often so poorly nourished that their operations had to be delayed until this could be corrected. It was found that patients fed intravenously not only gained weight, but also reported that their symptoms of diarrhoea and pain improved. When they returned to normal eating, however, they rapidly relapsed.

Intravenous feeding is potentially dangerous because of the risks of bacterial or fungal infection and liver failure. It was soon discovered, however, that elemental feeds were just as effective as intravenous nutrition in relieving the symptoms of CD. Elemental feeds had been developed by NASA for use in their space programmes for astronauts. They were pre-digested liquid foods whose contents were broken down to their simplest components – proteins to amino acids, starches to sugars, a single fatty oil, and minerals and vitamins added to make them nutritionally adequate. Despite being flavoured, they tasted dreadful at first! Nowadays the taste has greatly improved and the majority of patients can drink them with little difficulty.

Elemental feeds are highly effective in relieving CD. Such time away from normal eating does demand great determination, but the improvement of symptoms provides a strong incentive for the patient to continue.

HOW DOES DIETARY TREATMENT WORK?

There is still much discussion as to how elemental diet works in CD. It was initially suggested that it might allow the gut to rest, or that it improved nutrition, or that it removed food allergens from the diet. We now know that all these are only partially true, if at all.

We believe that elemental diet is effective because it deprives the bowel bacteria of the energy they require to thrive. Elemental diet is quickly and completely absorbed in the upper small intestine and little, if any, residue passes down to the lower gut where most bacteria live. After one week of elemental feeding the number of bacteria falls by over 50% and their activity is reduced. This results in a decline in the immune attack on the bacteria, thus symptoms dramatically improve.

When the patient's symptoms have settled, the elemental diet may be stopped. However, returning to a normal diet will lead to rapid relapse. The next stage in treatment involves the gradual reintroduction of normal foods in a carefully controlled manner so that any that provoke symptoms are identified and thereafter avoided. We believe specific foods stimulate bacterial activity and hence reactivate the disease. Unfortunately, these foods differ from patient to patient.

As already stated, in coeliac disease, 97% of patients respond successfully to a gluten-free diet, and treatment is therefore relatively simple. In CD, there is a range of foods that may be implicated. One patient may be upset by chocolate, another by wheat and gluten, another by milk. Likewise, the number of problem foods concerned may vary, from a single item to as many as a dozen.

The process of food reintroduction is therefore crucial to the success of the procedure and should be undertaken with the regular support and supervision of a dietitian, experienced in this field.

Following remission on elemental diet, the simplest way of reintroducing food is to start on an exclusion diet, similar to that which we have used with great success in patients with IBS. This is a balanced diet, avoiding those foods most frequently reported by CD sufferers to cause upset. Foods that are high in fat and fibre also commonly cause problems in CD and so these too are limited in the initial stages of the diet. The diet that we have developed is known as the LOFFLEX Diet (LOw Fat, Fibre Limited EXclusion diet). This allows the patient to switch straight from the elemental diet to a range of foods that rarely cause difficulties. If, after a further two weeks they are still feeling well, then the remaining foods are reintroduced slowly one by one in order to detect intolerances.

If symptoms recur on the basic LOFFLEX diet, it may be necessary to follow an elimination diet, a slower and more cumbersome procedure. Here, a single new food is reintroduced every day while the patient continues on elemental feeds until there are sufficient normal foods to allow a balanced diet. This may be a more successful method of reintroduction for a patient with unusual food intolerances, but we find that this method is not usually necessary for patients with CD. When the food reintroductions are complete, it is necessary for the dietitian to check the final diet to ensure that it is nutritionally adequate and to suggest ways of correcting any deficiencies.

Understandably, a number of patients struggle to complete such a demanding dietary programme. In our experience 25–30% are unable to continue on elemental diet long enough to reach remission. A further 10–15% drop out during the process of food reintroduction.

However, once food intolerances have been accurately established, relapse is unusual if the patient keeps to the diet.

We have found that nearly 60% of patients are still well two years after starting the diet with **no other treatment required**. It is most unusual for these patients subsequently to relapse, and after five years many find they can slowly return to normal eating as the CD appears to burn itself out. There are few, if any, side-effects.

We have shown that these patients do not develop thinning of the bones, and women can undergo normal pregnancies without changing their treatment. Perhaps most important of all, the patients feels in complete control of the CD and is able to ensure that it does not cause difficulties at crucial moments such as exams or holidays.

In CD, diet is effective only against active inflammation. It will not correct infection, previous damage to the bowel or the effects of surgery. There is no point in starting the diet if the disease is inactive. It is most important to check with your doctors that inflammation is the likely cause of your symptoms before setting out to try dietary treatment. Diet is NOT an effective treatment in active UC.

THE ELEMENTAL DIET AND LOFFLEX DIET

STAGE 1: ACHIEVING REMISSION ON THE ELEMENTAL DIET

If your doctor agrees that you should try diet as an appropriate treatment for your active CD, you will need to start off with a course of elemental feeds, which can only be obtained from your doctor. Dietary treatment will not be effective if you are on a high dose of corticosteroids and you will need to discuss with your doctor how gradually to reduce your medication before starting, or while you are taking, elemental feeds. Do not change any medication without your doctor's advice as this could potentially be very dangerous, especially if you are taking a corticosteroid. This is a type of hormone that your body produces normally, but in smaller amounts. When you are taking these pills, your body adapts to this supply and stops making the hormone itself. If you suddenly stop taking your medication, your body will not have time to turn on its own supplies again, leading to a hormone deficiency that can be very dangerous.

It is best to continue on other medication (apart from corticosteroids) until the disease is in full remission after dietary manipulation. There will be plenty of time to tail them off when you are well and reducing medication at the same time as starting elemental diet is sometimes over-ambitious.

Your doctor will refer you to a specially trained dietitian, who will advise you on how to take the elemental feeds. The dietitian will explain how much you will need to drink each day so as to reach or maintain a healthy weight. For the diet to succeed all other foods and drinks, apart from water, will be stopped. In our experience E028 Extra is very effective. This is available in liquid or powder form, flavoured or unflavoured. The powder is reconstituted by adding water. Another very successful feed is Pepdite 1+. This contains small strings of two or three amino acids and therefore has a lower osmotic pressure than E028. This means it draws less water into the gut and is less likely to cause diarrhoea. Many of the feeds available for treatment of CD contain too much fat. We only recommend feeds in which less than 15% of total energy is provided by fat (long chain triglycerides).

The elemental diet needs to be introduced slowly over a few days, gradually building up to the quantity recommended by your dietitian. It is best to sip the feed slowly through the day, rather than taking it only at mealtimes. The feed tastes better when chilled; some people like to eat it semi-frozen as a fruit slush. You may develop headaches during the first few days as your body gets used to the drink. This can be particularly noticeable if you are used to drinking a lot of tea or coffee and suffer caffeine withdrawal, but the headaches should soon pass. Make sure you drink plenty of water, especially in the early stages when you are building up the volume of elemental diet. If you need to take something to relieve these symptoms, remember to use *soluble* paracetamol and not tablets, which contain significant amounts of starches.

Some people feel nauseous at the start of the treatment. Drinking through a straw or diluting the feed with a little more water can help. However, do not dilute it so much that you struggle to consume the volume of elemental diet you need each day.

You will probably notice that your stools turn green and you develop bad breath. Don't worry. These are normal effects and show that the feed is working by reducing the activities of your bowel bacteria. Brushing your teeth more regularly will help improve your breath and these effects will soon clear when you get back to eating ordinary foods again.

Usually symptoms will have improved by around seven days, but it's essential that you complete the prescribed course in order to get the underlying inflammation properly under control. This usually takes between two to three weeks, although your doctor may advise you to continue for a little longer if your symptoms have not entirely settled at the end of this period. There is no point in starting the next stage of treatment if your disease is still active.

There are occasions, for example, after surgery or when patients are reasonably well controlled on medication, when we start nutritional treatment without using elemental diet. If symptoms are relatively few, it is permissible to go straight to the LOFFLEX diet for two weeks and then if all is well, to start the process of food testing.

STAGE 2: REINTRODUCING AND TESTING FOODS ON THE LOFFLEX DIET

By now you should be feeling very much better and longing to eat again. However, returning to a normal diet now will take you straight back to square one. To maintain remission from the disease, you must find out which foods are safe for you to eat and which are not. This can only be done by retesting foods individually to see which ones cause your symptoms to return. However, testing every single food would take a very long time. Having treated many patients with CD, we have found that there are a number of foods that rarely cause problems and therefore can be reintroduced into the diet straight away. These foods form the basis of the diet.

Fatty and high-fibre foods often upset patients with CD. As the liquid elemental diet is fibre-free and low in fat, it seems sensible to start on an exclusion diet with a reduced fat and fibre content and to increase these gradually to the individual's level of tolerance. For this reason, the exclusion diet we recommend for CD is the LOFFLEX diet. It is similar to that used in IBS, but the foods concerned are slightly different. Potato, for example, is sometimes a problem in IBS but rarely in CD. The foods that are allowed in the LOFFLEX diet and those that must be avoided are shown in the table below:

FOOD	NOT ALLOWED	ALLOWED
Meat	• pork • ham • bacon • meat products (e.g. sausages, beef burgers, pies, pâté and paste)	• all other lean meat and poultry (e.g. beef, lamb, chicken) – avoid all skin and visible fat
Fish	• fish in batter or crumb • fish tinned in oil or tomato • fish paste • taramasalata • scampi	• white fish • tinned tuna in brine • small portions of fatty, smoked and other tinned fish (in water or brine) • shellfish
Vegetables	• pulses (peas, beans, lentils) • onions • sweetcorn • tomatoes (incl. ketchup and purée, tinned veg in sauce e.g. baked beans)	• small portions of all other veg without skins, seeds or stalks – max. two portions daily
Fruit	• citrus fruit (e.g. oranges, grapefruit, lemons, satsumas) • apples • bananas • dried fruit and marmalade	• small portions of all other fruits, without skin or seeds, max. two portions per day fresh or cooked • jams free of orange/apple
Cereals	• wheat • oats • rye • corn • barley (check packet ingredients for this)	• white rice • rice pasta • rice cakes • puffed rice cereal • rice flour • ground rice • tapioca • sago • arrowroot

FOOD	NOT ALLOWED	ALLOWED
Cooking oils	• corn oil, vegetable oil, nut oil	(use sparingly: stir-fry only) • sunflower • soya • olive • rapeseed
Dairy products	• cow, goat, sheep milk and products (e.g. butter, margarine, cream, yoghurt, ice cream, cheese – check ingredients for these) • eggs	• soya milk and products (e.g. dairy-free margarine, soya yoghurt, cream and ice cream – small portions only as high fat) • tofu
Beverages	• tea • coffee (including decaf) • fruit squash • fizzy drinks • citrus, apple and tomato juice • all types of alcohol	• tap or mineral water, herbal and fruit teas (not containing citrus, fruit or apple), other fruit juices (e.g. pineapple, grape, black-currant)
Misc	• yeast (check ingredients) • salad cream and dressings • mustard • soy sauce • tinned and packet sauces • nuts • seeds • chocolate	• salt • pepper • herbs • spices (in moderation) • vinegar • sugar • honey • syrup • Kendal mint cake • carob

FOLLOWING THE LOFFLEX DIET

Here are some guidelines to help you follow the diet:

❭ Try to eat a wide variety of foods in the allowed list to help keep your diet balanced and interesting. You may find the sample menu below helpful. If you are struggling to find foods that you like, discuss this with your dietitian who may be able to suggest alternatives.

Breakfast – Rice cereal, soya milk, sugar/rice cakes, milk-free marg, honey and herbal tea

Light meal – Lean cooked red meat, chicken or fish, jacket potato (no skin), rice, rice cakes

Main meal – Lean cooked red meat, chicken, turkey or fish, potato, rice or rice pasta, cooked veg or salad, soya-milk-based dessert and portion of fruit

All the above suggestions are from the allowed list.

❭ Keep a food diary – a record of everything you eat throughout the day – and list any symptom you experience. This will help make it easier to identify any foods that you are intolerant to, even among those that are normally found to be safe. Buy a notebook and keep a double page for each day. On one side of the page write down all the foods you eat, and on the other the symptoms you notice. Record your bowel function and if you are a woman, your menstrual cycle. Remember to take the diary with you every time you go to see your doctor or dietitian!

❭ Keep in regular contact with your dietitian to discuss your progress. If you feel your symptoms are beginning to return, it is essential that you report this as soon as possible. Be honest with your dietitian if you are finding it a struggle sticking to the diet – let them know and a phone call should help to keep you motivated.

❯ If all remains well, after two weeks, your doctor and dietitian may feel you are ready to start reintroducing other foods into the diet. Do not start to do this until you have been given the go-ahead. Sometimes another week or two on the basic diet may be of benefit.

EXAMPLE OF A FOOD AND SYMPTOM DIARY

FOOD		SYMPTOMS
8 a.m.	**Breakfast** Rice Krispies, soya milk, sugar 2 rice cakes, soya margarine	9.00 a.m. diarrhoea
10.30 a.m.	banana, peppermint tea	
1 p.m.	**Lunch** grilled chicken, boiled rice, carrots pear, mineral water	2.30 p.m. abdominal pain
3 p.m.	rosehip tea	
6 p.m.	**Evening Meal** grilled cod, boiled potato, runner beans rice pudding made with soya milk camomile tea	7 p.m. bloating

REINTRODUCING FOODS

❯ Two weeks before starting the diet, record all the symptoms you have had and when, to help judge the value of the diet later on.

❯ For the first two weeks of the exclusion diet keep strictly to the list of allowed foods.

❯ During the third week you should eat as wide a variety of the allowed foods as possible. Each food should be tested for four days (and wheat for seven days). Include the test food at two separate meals or snacks each day or as indicated in the list below. If there is no reaction, the food can be kept in the diet and eaten in normal quantities. DONT FORGET TO KEEP YOUR FOOD AND SYMPTOM DIARY.

❯ If you react to a food, stop testing immediately. Do not continue testing for the full four days as this may cause your condition to relapse. Contact your dietitian and delay any further testing until you are fully recovered.

❯ If you have a particularly bad reaction to a food, you may need a short course of the elemental diet to settle your symptoms. You *must* discuss this with your dietitian and doctor. When you are ready to return to testing you do not need to start all over again from the beginning. Simply return to where you were in the list of reintroductions before you suffered the adverse reaction, obviously avoiding the problematic food.

❯ Foods that are high in fibre, e.g. oats, rye, banana, peas, wholegrain wheat, nuts, sweetcorn and barley, should be consumed in small portions on the first day, gradually increasing portion sizes over the remaining three days. If you notice an increase in discomfort or flatulence or your stools become looser, return to smaller portion sizes. Testing high-fibre foods this way will help you to discover whether the return of your symptoms is due to intolerance to the food itself or to the amount of fibre it contains. It should help you to determine a suitable level of fibre in your diet.

❯ Similarly, foods that are rich in fat, e.g. butter, margarine, chocolate and cheese, should be eaten in small amounts to begin with and then gradually increased as tolerated.

ORDER OF FOOD REINTRODUCTION

The order of reintroductions on the LOFFLEX diet is as follows:

Pork:	test as ham, bacon for snack meal and as roast, chop or mince for main
Oats:	test as porridge, oatcakes, flapjacks (check other ingredients)
Tea:	test x2 per day
Ryvita:	test at x2 meals per day
Eggs:	test at x2 meals per day
Onions:	test cooked and raw
Coffee:	test instant and real
Yeast:	take x3 brewer's yeast tablets, one at each meal
Banana:	test x2 per day
Apple:	test x2 per day

Milk:	test 560ml – 1pint – spread over the day
Butter/Marg:	test at all 3 meals
White wine:	test x2 glasses per day. If okay try red wine. If yeast not tolerated, try spirits (e.g. vodka, white rum)
Peas:	test x2 meals per day
Chocolate:	test as plain chocolate if milk not tolerated or as cocoa
Tomatoes:	test raw and cooked
Cheese:	test cooked and raw
Corn:	test as cornflakes and cornflour in cooking
Citrus fruit:	test oranges, grapefruit, satsumas or as fruit juice
Wheat:	test x7 days taking some at each meal
Yoghurt:	test at x2 meals per day, natural or flavoured
Nuts:	try different varieties 60g (2oz) per day
Sweetcorn:	small portions initially as very high fibre
Barley:	test barley flakes and pearl barley

When testing foods, it's important to remember that any unpleasant symptoms may indicate a reaction – it is not always the case that stomach pains or diarrhoea are the first symptoms to appear. During the period of food reintroduction, assume that all symptoms are caused by the food in question. However, symptoms may arise in other ways – as a result of picking up a bug or during the menstrual cycle, for example – and thus complicate the procedure. For this reason it is necessary to retest all foods that seem to trigger a reaction to make certain they are really the cause of the trouble. Leave a gap of two to three weeks before retesting a food that has upset you.

When you have completed all the testing, your dietitian will need to assess the nutritional adequacy of your final diet. You may be asked to complete an accurate diary of everything you eat and drink for a week. Analysis of your diary will indicate whether your diet is low in any of the essential nutrients. The dietitian can then advise you on which foods you could increase to improve the nutritional balance. It may also be necessary to supplement your diet with minerals or vitamins.

THE ELIMINATION DIET

Occasionally, patients may find that their disease goes into remission while on the elemental diet but as soon as they start the LOFFLEX diet they relapse straight away. This may be due to an undetected narrowing of the gut due to strictures. In this case the liquid diet will pass through without problems but any solid food will cause discomfort. Or it may indicate that a patient is intolerant to one or more of the 'safe' foods on the basic LOFFLEX diet. If further investigations rule out the presence of strictures, the patient can proceed with dietary treatment by introducing foods in a different way – known as the elimination diet.

This diet, unlike LOFFLEX, does not presume that any food is safe. Therefore, all foods have to be tested. This is obviously a more time-consuming approach and requires a patient to continue with elemental feeds until enough different foods have been reintroduced for the diet to be nutritionally balanced. Because the list of foods to be tested is so long, the testing period for each food is normally one day only. This can turn out to be too short, as some food reactions come on quite slowly. Therefore, it's sometimes better to slow the process of food testing.

This is particularly important when testing cereal grains and, as with the LOFFLEX diet, it is recommended that wheat is tested for seven days.

You must keep in regular contact with your dietitian and keep a detailed food and symptom diary. During the first two weeks the elemental diet can be gradually reduced, with the guidance of the dietitian. Foods being tested should be eaten at least twice per day and if no symptoms are experienced, can be taken in normal quantities thereafter. Foods that cause a reaction should be stopped immediately and further testing suspended until the patient is fully recovered. This may sometimes take several days. As with the LOFFLEX diet, elemental feeds may be required for a day or two to settle a particularly bad reaction.

The elimination diet below is based on the one I developed with the dietitians at Addenbrooke's Hospital.

Follow this order of food reintroduction on the days indicated. If you do not like a particular food simply leave it out and let your dietitian know.

> **NOTE:** All fruit and vegetables must be washed well.
> You may use salt, black pepper, herbs (not spices) for flavouring and also sugar, syrup and honey without testing them. You may drink herbal teas, e.g., camomile, peppermint, rosehip.

Test tap water for one day before starting food reintroductions.

THE ELIMINATION DIET: DAYS 1–9

DAY	FOOD	DESCRIPTION
Day 1	Chicken	Grill, steam, microwave or ovenbake in foil (do not add any fat)
Day 2	Rice	White or brown rice, boiled Rice cakes and Rice Krispies
Day 3	Pears	Raw, stewed or tinned in pear juice
Day 4	Milk free (soya) margarine	Use to cook chicken, spread on rice cakes and use in future cooking in moderation
Day 5	Soya milk	Not sweetened with apple juice
Day 6	Carrots	Fresh, frozen or tinned. Raw or boiled. Mash if desired
Day 7	Potatoes	Boiled, mashed, jacket or tinned. Potato flour may also be used
Days 8 & 9		Continue on safe foods from the first 7 days. If potatoes are not safe you could try sweet potatoes or eddoes once you have settled

MEAL PLAN (FROM DAY 7)

Omit those foods you cannot tolerate.

Breakfast	Rice Krispies with soya milk Potato cakes or rice cakes with milk-free margarine and honey Pear juice
Mid-morning	Rice cakes with honey
Snack meal	Cold chicken Grated carrot Rice cakes with milk-free margarine Pear
Main meal	Cooked chicken Mashed carrots with milk-free margarine Potatoes or rice Tinned pear or rice pudding made with soya milk
Supper	Pear juice Potato scones

THE ELIMINATION DIET: DAYS 10–19

DAY	FOOD	DESCRIPTION
Day 10	White fish	Cod, coley, haddock, monkfish, plaice, sole, whiting Grill with milk-free margarine or steam Try 2 types and if these are safe you may eat the others without testing them
Day 11	Runner beans	Fresh or frozen
Day 12	Cooking oil	(e.g. sunflower, rapeseed or olive) Do not use vegetable oil, which is a mix Use one type of oil only in small quantities (max. 1 tbsp per day)
Day 13	Bananas	Eat as a snack or add to Rice Krispies
Day 14	Turkey	Roast whole turkey, cook portions in the oven or use turkey pieces in a stir fry
Day 15	Peas	Fresh or frozen
Day 16	Milk	Whole, skimmed or semi-skimmed. Use on Rice Krispies, mashed potato, for rice pudding or as a drink Take at least 1 pint
Days 17 & 18		Continue on safe foods from the first 16 days
Day 19	Hard cheese	Cheddar/Edam/Cheshire

MEAL PLAN (FROM DAY 19)

Omit those foods you cannot tolerate.

Breakfast	Rice Krispies with milk Rice or potato cake with milk-free margarine and honey Pear juice
Mid-morning	Rice cakes with cheese
Snack meal	Cold chicken, turkey, carrot juice or home-made soup with allowed vegetables Rice salad (use cooked peas and carrots) Banana or pear Mineral water
Main meal	White fish cooked in milk or grilled Potatoes or rice Chicken or turkey risotto Runner beans and peas Rice pudding or stewed pears
Supper	Rice Krispies with milk and chopped banana Potato scones

THE ELIMINATION DIET: DAYS 20–30

DAY	FOOD	DESCRIPTION
Day 20	Tea	Ordinary tea with cow or soya milk
Day 21	Beef	Roast, casserole with allowed vegetables or use mince

DAY	FOOD	DESCRIPTION
Day 22	Apples	Wash skin well Bake or stew with sugar Also try apple juice
Day 23	Lamb	Roast a joint or grill chops You may also have lamb's liver
Day 24	Cauliflower	Fresh or frozen Wash well
Day 25	Tomatoes	Eat raw or grill Also try tinned tomatoes and tomato purée
Day 26	Mushrooms	Try grilled and raw or add to casseroles
Days 27	Eggs	Try boiled or fried
Day 28 & 29	Hard cheese	Continue on safe foods from the first 27 days. If eggs were safe, try scrambled eggs or omelette during the next 3 days If boiled or fried eggs are not tolerated you may still be able to use eggs in baking. Once wheat is tested try a quiche or cake containing eggs
Day 30		Butter or ordinary margarine

MEAL PLAN (FROM DAY 30)

Omit those foods you cannot tolerate.

Breakfast	Rice Krispies with milk Apple juice or tea
Mid-morning	Tea and rice cakes with margarine and cheese
Snack meal	Rice salad or rice cakes Raw carrot, mushroom and tomato Apple or banana Tea or apple juice
Main meal	Roast lamb, beef or chicken Potatoes Cauliflower, peas, carrots or beans Stewed apple, home-made meringue
Supper	Rice Krispies with milk and chopped banana Potato scones

Continue to add the following foods each day to extend your diet:

Spinach	Fresh or frozen
Oats	Test for 3 days Try porridge, oatcake biscuits or flapjack
Coffee	Test instant and ground coffee
Rye	Test as 6 Ryvita or other rye crispbreads If yeast is tolerated you could try 100% rye bread
Chocolate	Try plain chocolate bar (50g bar) and/or cocoa (3 tsps)

Barley	Test as pearl barley in soup or stew or barley flakes in muesli If barley upsets you, avoid malt
Beer/Lager	Test half a pint and if all well 1 pint the following day
Shellfish	Try prawns, shrimps, scampi, crab, lobster, mussels
Nuts	Test one 25g packet of one type of nut
Sweeteners	Test low-calorie drinks containing saccharin, aspartame and acesulphame K
Spirits	Test white spirits (e.g. vodka or white rum)
Wheat	Test for 7 days Try Weetabix, Shredded Wheat or wheat flakes Also pasta or wheat flour used with other ingredients already tested, e.g. to make biscuits or cakes
Yeast	Take 3 brewer's yeast tablets
Bread	Test white bread for 7 days only if you tolerated wheat and yeast
Fatty Fish	Herring, mackerel, pilchards, salmon, sardines or tuna Try fresh grilled or tinned in brine or suitable oil
Wine	Try white or red wine
Lettuce	Eat 2 large portions
Corn	Test for 4 days Try cornflakes, custard powder or cornflour Use cornflour to thicken sauces If these are tolerated try sweetcorn, popcorn or corn on the cob on the 4th day If you cannot take cornflour try arrowroot for thickening
Oil	Try corn oil or blended vegetable oil if corn is tolerated

Vinegar	Mix with oil and use as salad dressing, or put on chips
Pork	Test for 2 days Roast meat or grilled chop If this is tolerated try ham and bacon on the second day
Onion	Add to casseroles, stir fries, or mince Try raw in salads
Oranges	Test 2 oranges or 1 glass of orange juice Yoghurt (natural). Test 2 cartons per day

Now that you have tested a large number of foods you should be able to use many convenience foods. Check the ingredients and if it does not contain any foods you have not yet tested, or foods that have upset you, it may be included in your diet. You should also be able to eat out without too many problems.

So far you have not included many additives in your diet. These rarely cause a problem. As you use more convenience foods you will be including more additives. You do not need to test these but take a note of the additives in any foods which upset you and retest them again.

There are many fruits and vegetables still to test. These are listed below as a reminder to test each one. Continue to test only one food per day.

FOOD FAMILIES

Sometimes foods which are from related sources cross-react. Below are lists of foods which are from the same food families and which are therefore more likely to cross-react in this way.

Fruit

> Apricot, cherry, damson, greengage, nectarine, peach, plum, sloe
> Avocado pear
> White, red- and blackcurrants, gooseberry
> Blackberry, loganberry, raspberry
> Cranberry, bilberry
> Dried currants, grapes, raisins, sultanas
> Grapefruit, lemon, orange, tangerine, lime, kumquat
> Strawberry
> Pineapple

Nuts

> Almonds
> Brazil
> Cashew
> Chestnuts
> Coconut
> Hazelnuts
> Peanuts
> Pecans
> Pistachios
> Walnuts

Spices

> Chilli powder
> Cinnamon
> Coriander
> Cumin
> Curry powder
> Ginger
> Nutmeg
> Turmeric, etc

Vegetables

> Asparagus, leeks, garlic, chives, onions
> Artichoke (Jerusalem), sunflower seeds
> Aubergine, potato, tomato, peppers
> Beans (French, runner, butter, haricot, mung, kidney, beansprouts)
> Broad beans
> Beetroot, spinach
> Broccoli, cauliflower, mustard and cress, swede, turnip, spring greens, kale, Brussels sprouts, cabbage
> Celery, celeriac, parsnips, carrots
> Cucumber, gherkin, courgette, pumpkin, marrow
> Chicory, endive
> Lentils, soya beans

Continue to introduce foods each day taking three to four days to test oats, corn, rye and barley and seven days to test wheat. As in the LOFFLEX diet, gradually increase portion sizes of high-fibre cereals, veg and fruits to determine the level of fibre that is tolerated. When testing foods, it is important to remember that any unpleasant symptoms may indicate a reaction. During this period of food reintroduction, it should be assumed that all symptoms are caused by the food in question. Final diets must be assessed in the same way as the LOFFLEX diet to check that they are nutritionally complete.

KEEPING WELL ON YOUR DIET

It is important to remember that the diet you are following is an active treatment for a potentially dangerous disease and it must be continued if you wish to avoid a relapse. It is not possible to take a 'diet holiday'.

Many feel so well on their diets that they are tempted to believe that the CD has gone and they will be able to eat anything they like. Sadly, this is not true. You may find that you can get away with eating a problem food once maybe twice, but if you continue to eat it the disease will recur after a few days. Most patients find that five to ten years elapse before they can be really confident that problem foods no longer upset them. It is reasonable to re-test foods every year to make sure that they still cause trouble.

Sometimes it is difficult when travelling or visiting friends to avoid eating something that you know upsets you. If this happens, try to keep strictly to your diet for several days afterwards to allow the effects of this food to pass away. It is sensible always to have a small supply of elemental feed available in case of bad reactions, or if you get a gut upset perhaps from food poisoning or antibiotics. This will help prevent these setbacks developing into full relapses. When the symptoms subside, you will be able to go straight back to your previous diet.

IMMUNOSUPPRESSION IN THE TREATMENT OF CD

If you don't think that you can manage diet at this stage, then the alternative is immunosuppression.

As we are discussing the relative advantages and disadvantages of these treatments, it's fair to say that the remission rate with immunosuppressive drugs is less. Only 60–70% of people go into remission on corticosteroids, compared to 80–90% of those who are able to keep to elemental diet.

Immunosuppression does increase the risk of some nasty

problems, infections in particular. The nasty intra-abdominal abscesses that bedevil CD are nearly always seen in patients that have been given immunosuppression. Drugs such as infliximab increase the risk of tuberculosis. There may be other unpleasant side-effects such as osteoporosis or an increased risk of some forms of cancer. Furthermore, patients who have been given large doses of immunosuppressive drugs such as prednisolone are not good candidates for surgery. Anastamoses are more likely to break down and wounds to become infected. Surgeons much prefer to operate on patients who have not been receiving full doses of corticosteroids for several weeks beforehand.

On the other hand, immunosuppressive drugs are fairly simple to take, they involve little in the way of effort on the part of the patient and when they work, the response is very gratifying. Carefully managed, a regime such as prednisolone to induce remission, followed by an immunosuppressant such as azathioprine to maintain it, has worked well in many patients with CD who are very grateful for this treatment. At the end of the day, you are the most important person in deciding which treatment you would like. You must discuss this fully and in detail with your doctor. If your doctor appears not to support the course you would like to follow, then ask why you should not do so. If the explanation sounds unsatisfactory it is best to seek a second opinion because it's very important you are happy with the treatment you are offered.

Immunosuppression in CD is very similar to that used in UC (see chapter 6). The principle involved and the drugs used are the same. Thus powerful immunosuppressants such as corticosteroids or infliximab are given to induce remission and followed up by drugs such as 5-ASA, azathioprine, 6-MP or methotrexate to maintain remission in the long term. These drugs will be discussed in detail in chapter 6, which deals with the diet and treatment of patients with UC. There are, however, some drugs which are specifically used in CD, rather than UC.

Budesonide (Entocort, Budenofalk): a corticosteroid that was formerly introduced in the treatment of asthma, but which has a considerable advantage over prednisolone in that when it's taken orally 90% of it is destroyed in the liver, with only a small amount getting through into the systemic circulation. This of course means it produces fewer side-effects. It also means that its anti-inflammatory effect will be concentrated only on those parts of the gut where it is absorbed. If the drug is released in the small intestine, so little will pass through the liver that it will be ineffective in treating CD in the mouth or in the rectum, for example. Budesonide is therefore licensed for use in CD in the ileum and the ascending colon. It is supplied in capsules, which release 60–70% of its activity in this part of the gut. A small amount may reach further down the large intestine. It appears that although budesonide has fewer side-effects than prednisolone, unfortunately it may be less effective.

The usual dose for patients with ileo-caecal CD is 3mg by mouth three times per day. Budesonide is known to be valuable in acute mild to moderate CD, but its role in long-term maintenance is still not established. It is customary to give it in courses of up to eight weeks, tailing off the dose slightly before the dose is stopped completely.

Although the corticosteroid side-effects of budesonide are much less than other drugs in this group, nevertheless it is important to use it with caution in patients with tuberculosis, high blood pressure, diabetes, osteoporosis, glaucoma and cataracts or chicken pox or measles (see page 130–1). As yet there is little information of the value of budesonide in childhood CD and it's not known whether it passes into breast milk and whether it can be used in mothers who are breast-feeding.

Infliximab: this is a cytokine inhibitor. It stops the activity of tumour-necrosis factor alpha (TNF-α), which is a very powerful inflammatory cytokine. Cytokines are substances produced by white blood cells in response to infection and inflammation, and they may lead to tissue damage and ulceration. Infliximab is a monoclonal antibody, that is to say it has a very narrow target range and it binds and neutralises TNF-α. Infliximab is licensed for the treatment of moderate to severely active CD *not responding* to corticosteroids and or immunosuppressants.

One of the great advantages of infliximab is that it allows fistulae to heal. As we have seen fistulae may be difficult to treat and surgery to correct them is often fraught with difficulty. A course of infliximab may produce excellent results in over 50% of patients treated.

Unfortunately, infliximab is very expensive and this naturally deters doctors from using it freely. Private medical insurance companies are reluctant to pay for more than three infusions. Sometimes it is possible to be recruited into a medical trial at a nearby hospital to receive treatment without cost.

Infliximab is given as an infusion into a vein over about two hours. During this time you will be closely monitored in case of a possible reaction. The blood pressure, blood and temperature will be tested at half-hourly intervals throughout the infusion and one to two hourly intervals afterwards. The dose administered is calculated according to body weight and the most effective is 5mg per kg. Infliximab may be given as a single infusion or as three infusions repeated at two and six weeks after the initial dose. More recently it has been shown to be even more effective if it is given at regular intervals, approximately every eight weeks for a full year.

Infliximab, by blocking the effects of TNF-α, interrupts the chain of reactions leading to inflammation and tissue damage. Symptoms usually start to improve two to four weeks after treatment, and in approximately one-third of patients, full remission may be achieved after three infusions. Infliximab is used for inducing remission and it's customary to continue with immunosuppressive drugs such as azathioprine or methotrexate to prolong the remission afterwards. In some cases it may be necessary to continue with long-term infliximab to achieve optimum results.

Infliximab is a powerful drug which may have serious side-effects. It should not be given when there is liver or kidney damage or heart failure. TNF-α is normally part of the body's defence mechanisms; infliximab may increase susceptibility to infection. Latent tuberculosis may become reactivated and it's important that everyone who is being considered for treatment with this drug should first be tested for it. This is normally done by performing a T-spot test to look for circulating lymphocytes targeting tubercle bacteria, together with a chest X-ray. Infliximab may be associated with the development of abscesses related to the gut and infections in other parts of the body, including the brain. As the infliximab antibodies are derived partly from foreign proteins, they also may produce an allergic reaction. If so, treatment with infliximab will have to be stopped while they are dealt with. All patients need to be observed carefully for one to two hours after the infusion and resuscitation equipment has to be available for immediate use. Infliximab must only be administered in units where these facilities are available.

There is also a small risk of other side-effects including joint and muscle pains, rash, fever, itching, swelling of hands, face and lips, difficulty in swallowing and sore throat or headache.

Greater concern has been the suggestion that infliximab might increase the risk of cancer. It seems this is unlikely in

CD. For example, in one Italian study, 404 patients that were treated with infliximab were matched with 404 patients who never received it. Nine patients of the group who had had infliximab developed cancer, which was not significantly different from the control group where seven developed cancer. The age of diagnosis of cancer did not differ between the two groups. Similarly, no increased cancer risk or reduced survival in CD patients treated with infliximab was revealed in a US study, which followed up over 6,000 patients, despite the fact that the CD was more likely to be severe in those patients who were given infliximab. What's more, although the use of prednisolone more than doubled the risk of infection in this retrospective study, there appeared to be no additional risk of infection in patients treated with infliximab.

Adalimumab (Humira): another cytokine inhibitor that interferes with the action of TNF-α. However, it differs from infliximab as it does not need to be given intravenously, but can be given by a subcutaneous injection. Thus patients may administer it to themselves, as many diabetics do with insulin. Adalimumab is more effective than placebos in inducing remission in CD and 40% of patients, who went into remission, were still well 26 and 52 weeks later if they were continued on adalimumab treatment. It may reduce the dose of steroids required and help the healing of anal fistulae. It reduces rates of hospitalisation and surgery. It may also sometimes be effective in patients who are intolerant or unresponsive to infliximab. As many as 21% of patients in this group achieved remission on adalimumab and nearly half of them had some clinical response.

Like infliximab, adalimumab may increase the risk of infection and tuberculosis. There may again be severe allergic reactions. Common side-effects include back pain, headache, red and sore swelling of injection site, nausea, sinus inflammation and stomach pain.

More worrying side-effects include damage to the nervous system. There is a dose-dependent increased risk of malignancies in patients with rheumatoid arthritis treated with adalimumab, but it is not clear that this also applies to CD. A full list of side-effects by TNF-α antagonists is given at http://www.drugs.com/sitemap.html (then you can search for your particular drug). You must, of course, discuss treatment with any of these drugs fully with your doctor before you start any treatment so that any problems and anxieties can be allayed beforehand.

Natalizumab: a monoclonal antibody that stops the migration of white blood cells into inflamed tissue and thereby reduces the tissue damage. It has been shown to be significantly better than placebos for induction of a clinical response and remission in patients with moderately to severely active CD. In those studies, natalizumab was well tolerated. There have, however, been concerns that some patients treated this way developed a serious brain disease called progressive multi-focal leucoencephalopathy. The numbers of patients developing this condition was very small and the degree of risk involved in taking this drug is not yet clear. Currently this drug is only being used in specialist centres in patients who have failed to respond to TNF-α inhibitors.

The use of monoclonal antibodies to inhibit various components of the immune response is a topic of intense research at present and new drugs will no doubt soon be available. In all, it will be necessary to discuss carefully with your doctor the relative benefits that they are likely to provide in relation to the possible risks before deciding whether or not to go ahead with this treatment.

Other immune inhibitors: ciclosporin, mycophenolate

mofetil and tacrolimus are sometimes used in specialist centres (see page 135).

MAINTENANCE OF REMISSION IN CD

5-ASAs: frequently used to prevent relapse in CD and it's been shown in controlled trials that they are indeed effective. However, in my experience, they are relatively weak and although they may be very suitable in mild to moderate cases of CD, more severe cases usually need more powerful immunosuppressants.

Azathioprine: this is converted to 6-mercaptopurine (6-MP) in the body. These drugs are used most frequently to prolong remission in CD. They unfortunately produce side-effects in 20% of cases. These include suppression of the white cells and platelets, inflammation of the liver and pancreas and an increased risk of a form of cancer called lymphoma. Some patients develop malaise and fatigue, which makes continuing treatment unsuitable. Because of the risk of these side-effects, it's important that patients taking azathioprine or 6-mercaptopurine have a full blood count and liver function test done every two weeks during the first three months of treatment and at three-monthly intervals after that time. However, patients who have had side-effects on azathioprine may be able to take 6-mercaptopurine without their recurrence.

Patients metabolise these drugs at different rates and in some hospitals the enzyme involved (thiopurine S-methyltransferase – TPMT) is measured so that those with low levels can start on reduced doses. A new development which may be of great help in reducing the risk of side-effects is to give an enzyme inhibitor, allopurinol, together with a much reduced dose of azathioprine.

These drugs are less effective than corticosteroids at

producing remission of active CD and seem to take several weeks to work. It's therefore customary to cover their introduction by a course of corticosteroids, which should be tailed off as soon as remission is achieved.

It's clear that azathioprine and 6-MP will reduce disease recurrence over a period of six months to two years. What is not clear is how long after that treatment should continue.

I personally believe that it's important to keep disease in remission for as long as possible as this increases the chances of the condition burning itself out. However, one large retrospective study from France suggested that after four years of treatment, the risk of relapse was no greater in patients in which azathioprine had been withdrawn than it was in those that continued the drug, and for this reason many stopped at that stage. My own view is that if patients are well and suffering no ill-effects from the azathioprine, it's probably reasonable to continue with it, rather than risk further CD activity. However, there are reports of bone marrow damage even after several years' treatment and the relative risks of azathioprine and the likelihood of side-effects is something that you and your doctor must discuss in order that you are both happy with continuing treatment.

Methotrexate: this is indicated for maintaining remission in CD. A single dose of 20–25mg is given at weekly intervals. Because methotrexate depletes the body of folic acid, it is necessary to take a regular supplement. As with other immunomodulators, it's important to check for damage in the bone marrow and the liver in patients started on methotrexate should have weekly blood counts and kidney and liver function tests for the first two to three months and thereafter at three-monthly intervals.

Methotrexate should not be used in patients who have

kidney problems, and may cause gut upsets. This may first start with ulcers in the mouth or a sore throat, and such a symptom should be reported immediately to your doctor. Methotrexate may also cause cirrhosis of the liver and damage the lungs; aspirin and other NSAIDs should not be taken at the same time. Because methotrexate may damage an embryo in the womb, it is *essential* that women taking it should be on reliable contraception, which must be continued for three months after the drug has been withdrawn.

Sometimes in very difficult CD, methotrexate may be given by injection instead of by mouth.

TREATMENT OF COMPLICATIONS OF CD

The treatment described so far has been to control the acute inflammation of CD. CD may also cause a range of complications and their treatment is discussed in detail in chapter 7.

Immunosuppression is often highly effective in the management of CD. Furthermore, it can be used at the same time as nutritional treatment because the two are complementary: drugs reducing the activity of the immune system, and diet the activity of the colonic bacteria. The two together are sometimes invaluable in refractory cases, and have enabled many patients to avoid surgery. There is no single 'correct' way of treating CD – discuss the possibilities with your doctor, and choose the one that is right for you.

CHAPTER 6

Diet and treatment of ulcerative colitis

All the major drugs used in UC are only available on prescription. Your doctor will therefore decide which you will take. This is no place for self-treatment, but it is important that you understand the principles underlying your management and the drugs that are available as well as the relative benefits and disadvantages.

As we have seen (page 26) UC like CD involves an immune attack on the body by the bacteria resident in the bowel. The crucial difference between CD and UC is that in UC those bacteria appear to gain their energy requirements from substances normally present in the bowel rather than from food residues. It is therefore far more difficult in UC to modify the metabolism of the gut bacteria than it is in CD. Antibiotics may be helpful and probiotics hold great promise for the future (see page 228), but presently the treatment for UC is based largely on immunosuppression.

GENERAL MEASURES IN THE MANAGEMENT OF UC

Because the main symptom of UC is diarrhoea and because this is a very embarrassing and inconvenient symptom to suffer, there is a great temptation to take anti-diarrhoeal agents such as codeine, co-phenotrope (Lomotil) or loperamide (Imodium). This is usually a mistake. These drugs do not reduce the inflammation in the gut. Diarrhoea is one of the body's defence mechanisms – a way of getting rid of unwanted chemicals from the intestine. It certainly occurs after all manner of poisonings. Just read *Madame Bovary* for a graphic description! Furthermore, the number of stools you are passing is a reliable indication of just how bad your condition has become. If you regularly take anti-diarrhoeals, not only is the frequency of stool artificially reduced, giving a false impression of improvement, but also toxic chemicals produced by the gut bacteria are retained for longer in the body with the result that there is a greater risk of severe complications such as toxic megacolon and perforation. If the inflammatory process is being adequately controlled, diarrhoea will inevitably cease.

This is not to say that you should never take an anti-diarrhoeal tablet. There are occasions – an important meeting, or perhaps an exam – when a tablet of codeine may make all the difference between a confident perfor-mance and (literally!) gut-wringing anxiety. But *don't* do it regularly. Follow treatment that controls the inflammation rather than just stops diarrhoea.

CONSTIPATION

It is particularly important that patients with UC, espe-cially when it affects the left side of the bowel, avoid constipation as this is a factor that can lead to further relapses. The management of constipation is discussed on pages 145–147, 224. Follow this advice to try and prevent constipation setting in. In this way you may avoid relapses and the disappointment of having to go through a phase of treatment yet again.

NICOTINE

As it's been shown that patients who smoke are less likely to have a relapse of their colitis, it's been suggested that nicotine might be an effective treatment for the condition. A number of trials have been carried out in which nicotine has been administered in various ways (e.g. skin patches, chewing gum) and in some of these there were positive results: patients treated with nicotine did better than those given a placebo. However, the improvement was not dramatic and there were other side-effects. Nicotine therefore does not appear to represent a dramatic improvement in the management of UC. There is still uncertainty about how smoking helps patients with UC. People who have smoked will know that an early morning cigarette often has a noticeable laxative effect and the benefits of smoking may be no more than taking a suitable laxative. (See pages 39, 203 for further details on smoking.)

CONTROL OF INTESTINAL INFLAMMATION

The basic plan of action is to suppress the immune attack on the gut bacteria by using a powerful agent such as corticosteroids, ciclosporine or infliximab and at the same time to start treatment with an agent which may be continued in the long term to keep the disease under control without damaging side-effects, thus allowing the first agent to be tailed off. Drugs used in UC may therefore be divided into two groups: agents that induce remission and those that maintain remission.

AGENTS THAT INDUCE REMISSION

Corticosteroids (prednisolone, hydrocortisone, methyl prednisolone): cortisol (hydrocortisone) is a hormone produced by the adrenal glands, which lie in the abdominal cavity just above the kidneys. It is crucial to the maintenance of water, sodium and potassium balance in the body, and is essential for life. A number of chemicals with a similar chemical structure and physiological effects have now been synthesised, and are used in medicine, being known collectively as 'corticosteroids'. Corticosteroids are often referred to as 'steroids', but this can be confusing as a number of other preparations are available which also share a common steroid chemical structure. The contraceptive pill, for example, is comprised of steroid hormones, and anabolic steroids, which may be used to build up muscle bulk and strength, have developed a bad reputation because they have often been taken by athletes to improve their performance artificially. Thus, though your doctor and nurses may frequently refer to 'steroids', in this book I prefer to use the full description 'corticosteroids' to avoid any confusion.

The introduction of corticosteroids into the treatment of UC was a dramatic step forward. In former days, it was not uncommon for patients to die from severe colitis and the introduction of corticosteroids cut death rates dramatically. Nowadays, patients with UC have virtually the same life expectancy as the general population. Nevertheless, initial enthusiasm soon became tempered by the realisation that corticosteroids may have important side-effects.

This is because, in addition to their immunosuppressive effect, corticosteroids, just like the hormones produced by the adrenal glands, have dramatic effects on the body's metabolism. They act on the kidney to cause conservation of sodium by the body, with increased losses of potassium.

They promote the production of sugar by increasing the breakdown of protein to glucose, and they may also have an effect akin to a steroid sex hormone and increase the growth of body hair.

The effect of reducing sodium excretion by the kidneys means that body fluids are increased. This may cause mild swelling of the ankles and it may also lead to an increase in blood pressure. Increased pressure in the eyes may trigger glaucoma. Loss of potassium from the body may cause muscular weakness.

The breakdown of protein to form extra sugar may lead to the development of diabetes in susceptible people. The extra sugar tends to get laid down as fat around the body, leading to obesity. At the same time the loss of protein weakens many tissues in the body. The most important of these is bone, where the loss of protein leads to osteoporosis. However, protein is also lost from the skin which tends to become thinner with the development of scars knows as striae. Loss of protein from the muscles makes them smaller and weaker and loss of protein from the blood vessels makes them more likely to burst causing dark bruises known as purpura under the skin. The combination of all these effects – a fatty face and body because of increased sugar production and thin arms and legs because of loss of muscle bulk – has led to the effects of prolonged corticosteroids administration being described as a 'lemon on sticks'.

Corticosteroids may also produce mental disturbances. Some become very overactive and unable to settle and relax. Many patients have difficulty in sleeping and a very few develop serious mental problems such as paranoia and depression. Clearly the amount of corticosteroids given must be kept as low as possible.

In order to obtain the therapeutic benefit of corticosteroids with the fewest possible side-effects, it has become common to use them in preparations, which are applied only at the site of inflammation. This is known as topical treatment. Several preparations are available which can be applied through the anus and which will flow along the bowel to cover all the area which is inflamed. Corticosteroid suppositories can be inserted just inside the anus to treat proctitis. Foams are valuable in proctosigmoiditis, and if used correctly enemas will reach as high as the splenic flexure, thus being of great value in left-sided colitis.

In severe cases of UC, however, the drug needs to be given systemically – that is to say either by mouth or injection. In both cases it spreads throughout the body and is most likely to have side-effects. Nevertheless, in severe cases of acute UC intravenous or oral corticosteroids are often lifesaving.

The main preparations of corticosteroids available are as follows:

❯ **Suppositories** (Predsol): a bullet-shaped tablet that is pressed through the anus into the rectum. There the warmth of the body allows it to melt and the drug is gradually absorbed into the mucosa. The drug does not spread far up the bowel and so suppositories are most suitable for use in proctitis. However, they may also be valuable in patients with left-sided colitis if they are given half an hour before an enema. This may produce a soothing effect, which allows the enema to be retained in the bowel for longer and thus have better therapeutic value.

❯ **Foam enema** (Predfoam, Colifoam): these are contained in small pressurised containers which have a tube attached. The tube is passed through the anus into the rectum and a press of the button releases the necessary amount of foam. Foam has the advantage that it is retained in the bowel more easily than liquid, but it does not reach as high so is best used in inflammation affecting just the rectum and sigmoid.

❱ **Liquid enemas** (Pred Enema or Predsol): when UC extends up to the left side of the colon, it may be treated by a liquid steroid enema. These enemas come in a bag containing a liquid corticosteroid. There is a tube attached which is passed through the anus into the bowel. The bag is slowly squeezed by hand so that a gentle stream of liquid enters the rectum. Obviously, with a liquid there is the potential for leakage, but this can be avoided with practice. Liquid enemas are usually given at night and ideally are retained as long as possible, even until the next morning. If you lie on your face with a pillow under your hips, it will raise the buttocks and the liquid will run under the influence of gravity, up the bowel towards the splenic flexure. Some people find that it is difficult to retain the liquid, particularly if they are producing lots of wind, and they may have to rush off to the loo before the enema can have its full therapeutic effect. As mentioned earlier, putting a suppository in 30 minutes earlier may help with this problem.

It is usual to treat distal UC with suppositories or enemas for two to four weeks. If at the end of that time the condition has not improved, something different is tried.

❱ **Oral corticosteroids:** in Britain, prednisolone is the most widely used oral form of corticosteroid, but sometimes other preparations such as hydrocortisone or methyl prednisolone are substituted. It is customary to start with a high dose of up to 60mg daily, preferably taken in the morning after breakfast. When the drug starts to work, the dose can be tailed down, and ideally stopped altogether. Unfortunately, corticosteroids are not an efficient way of prolonging remission – most trials have been negative.

All patients who are taking systemic corticosteroids should carry a 'steroid card'. This gives their name and other personal details, together with the dose of corticosteroid being taken and the date the course started. This is because stopping corticosteroids abruptly may be dangerous. The production of corticosteroid hormones in the body is carefully controlled by the pituitary gland. When therapeutic doses of corticosteroids are given, as in UC, for three weeks or longer, the pituitary gland may switch off. Under these circumstances it is very dangerous to stop corticosteroids suddenly as the patient's own adrenal glands may have shut down because of the lack of any drive from the pituitary and stopped producing their hormones. There may be a gap before they restart. Lack of cortisol may lead to serious problems – weakness, vomiting and low blood pressure – and if a patient were unconscious or confused after an accident, he might not be in a fit condition to tell doctors about his corticosteroid treatment.

Patients who have received previous courses of corticosteroids in the previous year, or who have received doses of more than 40mg a day, are also at risk of this adrenal suppression even when the duration of the present course of treatment may be less than three weeks. It is always safer to tail the dose off gradually.

Intravenous preparations of steroids act most quickly of all. When UC is so severe that hospital admission is required, it's often decided to give corticosteroids in this way but as soon as the patient starts to respond to the intravenous steroids it's customary to switch over to tablets by mouth.

OTHER DRUGS TO INDUCE REMISSION

Ciclosporin: this was introduced for use in organ transplantation but is sometimes necessary in severe cases of UC that do not appear to be responding to corticosteroids. Thus it is only used in severe cases of pancolitis admitted for treatment in hospital. It may damage the kidneys, and treatment, which starts intravenously, must be monitored very carefully with measurement of the blood levels of the drug and kidney function tests. It may cause high blood pressure. If the initial response is favourable, the patients may be switched to an oral preparation, which may slowly be tailed off in the next few weeks. As with other immuno-suppressants, there is an increased risk of contracting infections.

Infliximab: this was introduced for the treatment of CD, but has how been shown to be helpful as an alternative in some cases of severe UC who might otherwise be given intravenous ciclosporin. Its use and its side-effects are discussed under the treatment of CD (page 120).

Other immunosuppressants sometimes used in specialist centres include tacrolimus and thalidomide. If treatment with either of these is suggested you should discuss the possible benefits and disadvantages carefully with your doctor.

Aminosalicylates: while drugs in this group are most commonly used maintain remission, they may sometimes be used to induce remission in mild to moderate cases of

UC, especially topically in cases of distal UC, a situation in which they are often highly effective (see page 133).

Acetarsol: this is a substance derived from arsenic. However, although arsenic is poisonous, acetarsol has been found to be very effective in cases of resistant proctitis. In clearly defined doses it is safe and effective. Acetarsol is used only in refractory distal colitis that has failed to respond to steroids and 5-ASA. The dose is usually 2x 50mg suppositories once or twice a day for up to four weeks. The suppositories should be lubricated with a little gel before insertion into the rectum. Side-effects are few and far between. Some cases of poisoning have occurred with prolonged courses (more than four years in both cases) or when large doses totalling 3.5 to 7.9g, the level in the blood and urine may initially be high, but usually falls after the week as the lining of the rectum heals and reduces arsenic absorption. After four weeks, when treatment ceases, there should be no residual arsenic in the blood.

Acetarsol is not listed in recent copies of the *British National Formulary* and may have to be supplied by special order through hospital pharmacies, which may not always be possible.

DRUGS TO MAINTAIN REMISSION

Aminosalicylates (Salazopyrin, Asacol, Ipocol, Mesren, Pentasa, Salofalk, Dipentum and Colazide): the drugs most commonly prescribed for keeping UC in remission. They reduce inflammation by complex mechanisms, which are still not completely understood. As they are related to aspirin they should not be taken by patients who are allergic to it.

Sulphasalazine (Salazopyrin) was the first drug in this group to be discovered, as long ago as 1942. It was first developed for the treatment of rheumatoid arthritis and indeed is still widely used for this purpose, but when it was given to a patient with arthritis related to UC it was found that his bowels improved even more than his joints! Since then it has been widely used in the treatment of IBD. Unfortunately, it produces side-effects in as many as 25% of people taking it. These include nausea and vomiting, which was reduced by adminstering it in enteric-coated capsules which prevent release in the stomach. It may also depress the bone marrow, cause very nasty skin rashes and damage the liver and kidneys. It increases the breakdown of red cells in certain people who are deficient in an enzyme called glucose 6-phosphate dehydrogenase (G6PD).

These effects naturally caused great anxiety and led to more research. It was then discovered that, in the bowel, sulphasalazine is broken down into two separate compounds – sulphapyridine which is largely excreted in the urine turning it very yellow, and 5-aminosalicylic acid (5-ASA). The side-effects were caused mostly by the sulphapyridine, while the 5-ASA had the therapeutic effect. Unfortunately, since 5-ASA is broken down in the upper gut, it is necessary to find some way of getting it down to the scene of the action before it has been destroyed. It has to be delivered in various ingenious ways enabling the active drug to be released in the colon. Many of these depend on binding it to resins, which release it at a pre-determined level of acidity (pH). It's therefore important to avoid medicines that may change the pH of the colon. Lactulose, for example, makes the colon slightly more acidic and this may interfere with the release of 5-ASA from some preparations.

Although none of these 5-ASA preparations contain sulphapyridine, they do sometimes have side-effects. If you develop any unexplained bleeding (other than from the bowel), bruising, sore throat, fever or malaise, you should let your doctor know immediately. Sometimes 5-ASA makes diarrhoea worse. This is particularly true of olsalazine, which contains two molecules of 5-ASA. This means that it is often more effective, but it is wise to build up the dose slowly, starting with a single capsule daily, and increasing the dose by one capsule every few days until the desired level is reached.

It's also important to check each year that 5-ASA is not damaging your kidneys – a simple blood test by your GP is all that is necessary.

As there are several drugs available in this group, if one does not work, it's usual to try another. I generally start my patient on one of the forms of mesalazine (Asacol, Pentasa) and if this is not adequately effective, I change it in the first place to olsalazine (Dipentum).

Mesalazine is also available in topical form – suppositories and enemas. When remission has been induced with topical 5-ASA, it is usual to switch to oral forms to maintain remission. Far easier to swallow a pill than insert an enema!

There is no general agreement on how long 5-ASA therapy should continue in patients who are in remission. Many wish to stop treatment once they are better. I believe that this just leads to early relapse and I like to continue in the hope that the disease may burn itself out. However, it is always difficult to know when this has happened. I generally ask my patients to continue 5-ASA for three years after their last relapse before stopping it. If they then relapse, they start another three-year stint.

IMMUNOSUPPRESSANTS

Most patients with UC are initially treated by a combination of a corticosteroid with 5-ASA. When this combination does not prevent further relapses, it's usual to try adding an immunosuppressant.

The two most commonly used are azathioprine (Imuran) and 6-mercaptopurine (Puri-nethol). These are very closely related; indeed azathioprine is converted to 6-mercaptopurine (6-MP) in the body. These are now accepted as being an excellent treatment for UC. Unfortunately, it takes several weeks, sometimes up to three months, for them to be fully effective. It's customary, therefore, to cover their introduction with a further course of corticosteroids. In many cases the 'steroid sparing effect' of azathioprine or 6-MP allows the corticosteroids to be tailed off completely. If necessary, 5-ASA can be continued at the same time as the immunosuppressant.

People vary in their capacity to metabolise azathioprine and 6-MP. It's now possible to measure the enzyme responsible for this, which is called thiopurine S-methyltransferase (TPMT). If the level of the enzyme is low, a therapeutic effect can be achieved with a smaller dose of drug. Nevertheless many doctors feel that such a test is unnecessary. They start their patients on a small dose and if, after four weeks have elapsed, there are no ill-effects, increase to the full therapeutic dose, which is 2–2.5mg azathioprine or 2.5mg 6-MP per kg body weight.

The main disadvantage of azathioprine and 6-MP is their side-effects. These may affect as many as 20% of patients, but it seems that the risk is less with 6-MP than with azathioprine itself, even though azathioprine is converted to 6-MP in the body. Be that as it may, it is vital that full blood count and liver function tests are done every two weeks for the first two months of treatment and then every three months to see if the drugs are damaging the bone marrow or the liver. They may sometimes also affect the pancreas. In a number of patients there is no specific effect on any organ, but they experience an overwhelming feeling of malaise and fatigue, which also means that the drug has to be abandoned.

After three months, if all is well, it's possible to reduce the frequency of these tests to every three months. However, if at any stage the dose of azathioprine or 6-MP is increased, it's sensible to go through weekly testing for three months yet again. Remember: these drugs may have a wonderfully beneficial effect on your UC, but that doesn't mean they will always be safe. Never forget to go along for your blood tests!

When there are no side-effects, however, there can be no doubt that this group of drugs are of tremendous value in keeping patients in remission and off steroids. The difficulty is to know how long to continue them. A French study a few years ago suggested that after four years there was no advantage in keeping them going, but we sometimes find that UC relapses when the drug is withdrawn even in patients who have been on them for so long. This is something to discuss with your doctors.

OTHER DRUGS TO MAINTAIN REMISSION

Other drugs that may be used occasionally to maintain remission, usually in patients who have been upset by azathioprine, or 6-MP, include:

Methotrexate: this is taken once a week together with folic acid to prevent side-effects (see page 125).

Mycophenolate mofetil: this again is a powerful immuno-suppressant introduced in transplantation whose side-effects mean that careful monitoring must always been undertaken. If it's suggested that you try one of these drugs, you must discuss the matter fully with your doctor beforehand.

TREATMENT OF INDETERMINATE COLITIS

I usually recommend that indeterminate colitis be treated in exactly the same way as UC itself. The patchy colonic inflammation raises echoes of CD, but in my experience diet is rarely successful. In some cases there is initial improvement, but after a few months relapse inevitably occurs, and does not respond to a further course of elemental diet. Perhaps the bacteria involved here are initially capable of obtaining energy from either food residues or endogenous substrates in the bowel, but when the food residues are withdrawn they switch over to colonic sources alone – and the condition becomes straightforward ulcerative colitis! Fortunately results are generally rather good.

DIET IN UC

You have seen that I am clearly a great enthusiast for the use of diet to treat CD! It may therefore seem surprising that I am quite clear that diet does not play a therapeutic role in UC. There was excitement in the 1960s when researchers in Oxford reported that they had successfully treated some patients with UC by means of a milk-free diet. Because of this work, some gastroenterologists recommend milk-free diets for UC patients even to this very day! A number of patients with UC may also suffer from alactasia, where there is a lack of the enzyme lactase in the lining of the small bowel. This enzyme splits the milk sugar lactose into glucose and galactose, which are then absorbed into the body. If the enzyme is missing, the lactose cannot be digested and passes down to the bacteria in the large bowel where it may precipitate flatulence and diarrhoea. This can obviously make UC symptoms worse.

However, I have yet to achieve genuine remission in any patient with UC by means of diet. At one stage I treated 16 successive patients with UC by feeding them intravenously. The role of diet in CD was first demonstrated when surgeons gave poorly nourished patients TPN (total parenteral nutrition) to build them up before their operations and get them fit for surgery. Intravenous feeding improved not only their state of nutrition, but also greatly reduced the amount of inflammation produced by the CD itself. The treatment of severe UC is often difficult and these patients too may be malnourished. Therefore, I felt it was quite reasonable to feed them intravenously to build them up and, at the back of my mind, I also hoped that it might also possibly, as with the CD patients, reduce the level of inflammation.

The patients were fed intravenously for 10–14 days and all of them still needed to have intravenous corticosteroids to bring the disease into remission. Some of them had to go on to surgery. Although this was not a formal controlled trial, it was quite clear to me that the intravenous feeding was not producing any benefit in terms of reducing inflammation.

In the 1960s it was thought that CD was a disease that affected the small bowel and only since then have we appreciated that it is possible to have CD in the large intestine alone. I suspect that the patients treated in Oxford were cases of colonic CD, which will, of course, respond favourably to diet. When UC and CD are so similar in so many ways, it may seem paradoxical that one should respond to diet and the other should not. Recent research on the action of elemental diet provides a possible explanation.

We now know (page 96) that bacterial fermentation changes in patients who are given elemental diet. Their stools turn green and chemicals such as phenols and indoles, which are not normally present, appear on the breath. When we gave elemental diet to normal volunteers, the number of bacteria present in the faeces dropped to 40% of the original level, showing that many had died. It is clear that for many bacteria living in the large intestine, food residues coming down from the small bowel are an important source of food.

However, some bacteria in the bowel depend not on food but on other substances in the bowel for their energy. Recently we had a clear demonstration of this when, together with colleagues from Birmingham University, we were looking at two types of bacteria which we thought were important in IBD. These were *Faecalibacterium prausnitzii* (Fp) which had been suggested to be present in reduced numbers in CD, and sulphate-reducing bacteria (SRBs) which have been suggested to be important in UC. We put a number of patients with active CD on elemental diet so that their symptoms subsided. We found, rather to our surprise, that there was plenty of Fp present in the stools before the elemental treatment was started, but that two weeks later, when their symptoms had improved considerably, the levels of this bacterium had fallen significantly.

Indeed, there was a significant relationship between the fall in numbers of Fp and how much the patient improved. Clearly Fp was dependent on normal food residues for its energy supplies. With the SRBs, however, we discovered a completely different picture. Levels of SRBs varied to a certain extent at the start of treatment, but by the end of treatment they had increased. Obviously these bacteria were living on something else and their numbers could increase even when no food residue was available.

This is not to claim, of course, that SRBs are the cause of UC. It merely shows that various bacteria have various sources of energy and the numbers of some will therefore not be affected by enteral feeding. It seems quite possible that the bacteria that trigger off the immune attack in UC get most of their energy substrates from breaking down mucus.

Mucus is the natural lubricant for the large intestine. It contains considerable amounts of sulphate, which could possibly be a source of nutrition for SRBs, but it is mainly composed of complex molecules of protein and carbohydrate. There is no doubt that it can provide suitable nutrients for a number of bacteria. If mucus was the source of energy for bacteria underlying UC, it would explain a number of features of the disease. There is much more mucus in the large bowel than in the small and this would explain why UC is limited to the colon. It would also explain why biopsies in UC – but not CD – show depletion of the mucus stores and why mucus from the bowel of patients with UC differs in chemical structure from that of people with normal bowels or those with CD. Lack of mucus deep in the bowel wall would explain why deep ulcers do not form in UC and, of course, bacteria, whose energy source was mucus, would not be affected in the least by feeding with elemental diet.

Thus it's not possible to control UC by modifying the diet. This does not mean that diet is unimportant in UC; on the contrary it is often crucial for maintaining nutrition, promoting normal gut function and preventing certain complications.

NUTRITION

Patients with UC may become malnourished. The illness may make them reluctant to eat, as eating often stimulates bowel activity. Inflammation in the bowel causes loss of blood and mucus, which can give rise to anaemia. Some of the drugs used may reduce the absorption of certain nutrients. Sulphasalazine reduces the absorption of folic acid, and corticosteroids need to be supplemented with calcium. Diarrhoea, by speeding the passage of food items down the gut, may also reduce their absorption and lead to malnourishment.

It's therefore important to eat regularly. Smaller meals are easier for the gut to deal with. It's better to eat less food more frequently, having perhaps six meals per day. If you have a greater variety of foods in your diet, it will become more interesting, but remember that there really are no foods in particular that patients with UC should avoid. If you need help, you should ask your doctor to send you to a registered dietitian.

Obviously you must work with your doctor to try and bring the disease under control. If you are feeling well, you will feel more like eating and the food will be better absorbed. Finally supplements may be required. Iron, calcium and folic acid are ones which are sometimes in short supply.

ROUGHAGE

The bowels do not work well unless the muscles that push the stools along have something to work on. Roughage is a general term for the indigestible food residues that pass into the faeces. A lot of the material is complex carbohydrates from plants, which may be referred to as fibre. Increasing roughage helps to make the stools bigger and softer so that they pass more easily along the bowel. If you don't have enough roughage you tend to be constipated, and if you have too much there may be a tendency to diarrhoea.

In general this roughage is very good for you. It reduces the amount of cholesterol in the blood and reduces the risk of developing gallstones, piles and diverticular disease. However, with UC patients it may increase the tendency to diarrhoea. Some patients are advised to reduce the amount of roughage in their diet to prevent a blockage at a stricture, and this may lead to constipation. A further problem is that some types of roughage may be fermented by the gut bacteria to produce excess gas and this may lead to bloating and discomfort. The type of fibre that you take is therefore important.

As I believe that constipation is a factor that makes it more likely that UC will relapse, I like my patients to take plenty of roughage, but on the other hand I prefer that this is not fermented to produce unpleasant flatulence. I often recommend that they supplement their diets with a bulking agent that is not amenable to fermentation. There are three of these, which are: cracked linseed, sterculia and methyl cellulose. They are invaluable for maintaining a regular bowel habit in patients with UC. Because they are not fermented they can be given at the same time as a diet low in other forms of fermentable fibre. In this way it is possible to reduce wind without causing constipation.

All forms of roughage absorb water; indeed, without this they would not be effective as bulking agents. It is therefore important that you drink plenty of water at the same time as making sure there is an adequate amount of roughage in your diet.

PROXIMAL CONSTIPATION

Patients with proctitis or left-sided colitis sometimes develop constipation higher up the larger intestine, that is to say on the right-hand side of the bowel. The doctor or nurse may be able to feel the bowel like a length of rope on the right side of the belly, or it may be demonstrated on an abdominal X-ray. Why this should be is not quite understood, but often we find we cannot get the inflammation to settle until the proximal constipation is cleared.

A high-roughage diet will help reduce the chances of proximal constipation developing. When it is present, however, it has to be flushed out using a purge such as Picolax or Citromag followed up by a laxative regime which usually comprises non-fermentable bulk laxatives such as cracked linseed or Normacol, with sometimes an occasional dose of syrup of figs or senna as well.

Food intolerance

Proximal constipation may also sometimes be due to food intolerances. Many people get mixed up between food allergy and food intolerance. In food allergy there are circulating antibodies in the blood, which will combine with the allergen to precipitate an allergic response. This can be comparatively mild and merely produce spots and itching, or sometimes it can be severe and dangerous, as for example when peanut allergy leads to swelling of the tongue and lips and can cause choking. Food allergies can be diagnosed by tests to show the relevant antibodies circulating in the blood.

Food intolerance is quite different. In this there are no circulating antibodies, and reactions do not come on quickly but fairly slowly. We now know that many of them are due to the changes to the balance of the bacteria in the colon. This changes fermentation of foods coming down the bowel so that they produce toxic chemicals that upset the bowel function.

As mentioned earlier, in UC the balance of bacteria in the large intestine is abnormal and the disease is also associated with a similar bacterial imbalance. It is not surprising therefore that patients with UC quite often have food intolerances similar to those seen in IBS. Many patients with UC find that if they eat certain foods they may get wind, pain or diarrhoea and it is not surprising they think these foods may be making their UC worse!

However, if they avoid the offending foods, it does *not* allow the UC to heal and medication is still necessary. Obviously, if you find a food upsets you, you should avoid it, but don't make the mistake of thinking that this will allow your UC to heal. Sometimes patients continue to suffer mild bowel symptoms even when their sigmoidoscopy shows that the lining of the bowel has healed. Under these circumstances, it is sensible to try an exclusion diet to identify any food intolerances (my book *Irritable Bowel Solutions*, Vermilion, 2007, gives full details of how this should be done) to see if this clears the matter.

If you continue to suffer difficulties because of persistent proximal constipation, it may again be well worth trying an exclusion diet, which is often successful in relieving the problem.

THE TREATMENT OF ULCERATIVE COLITIS: A SUMMARY

The above account of all the drugs available that can be used in the treatment of UC may lead to considerable confusion for patients. With so many to choose from, which is right for my case? Here, therefore is a brief summary of how they are generally applied in day-to-day practice at the present time. It is based on the recommendations of the American College of Gastroenterology (see *American Journal of Gastroenterology*, 2010, 105 501–23).

For **left-sided disease** and **proctitis**, mesalazine enemas and suppositories are used, and are more effective than topical steroids. Results are better if mesalazine is also given by mouth at the same time. Maintenance of remission can be achieved with mesalazine, either by mouth or as suppositories.

Extensive **colitis** is usually initially managed by high doses of oral sulphasalazine or mesalazine, keeping corticosteroids in reserve for refractory patients. Azathioprine or 6-mercaptopurine are used when patients do not respond to steroids, and are also used to get steroid doses down, and to maintain remission afterwards.

Patients with **severe refractory colitis** may require hospitalisation, especially if they have fever, a rapid pulse and low levels of albumin in the blood. They will need intravenous steroids, or, nowadays, infliximab. If improvement does not occur after three to five days, ciclosporin may be tried, but there also needs to be consideration of whether or not surgery to remove the large bowel would be advisable. Long-term remission after an initial response in this group is enhanced by adding 6-mercaptopurine or azathioprine, but the long-term efficacy of infliximab in these patients is not yet clear. Antibiotics – metronidazole or ciprofloxacin – are generally reserved for pouchitis (see page 187).

Not everything in medicine, of course, goes completely to plan and the above scheme is simply an outline of current practice. Your gastroenterologist may well advise something different if the first-line drugs are not sufficiently effective.

CHAPTER 7

Complications of IBD

IBD is, of course, primarily a disorder of the gut. Even when it first presents with problems in other organs such as the eye or the liver, inflammation will be detectable somewhere in the intestine even if at that stage it is not producing any symptoms. Certain complications, however, arise directly as a result of inflammation in the gut.

Anaemia: inflammation and ulceration of the gut lining leads to chronic bleeding into the intestine. This blood will be lost from the body and deplete the body's store of iron leading to an iron deficiency – anaemia. If the small bowel is damaged there may also be a failure to absorb folic acid and vitamin B12. Deficiency of these vitamins may lead to anaemia.

Anaemia causes tiredness. It can easily be checked by a simple blood test, which will show how much of the oxygen-carrying pigment, haemoglobin, is present. The blood test will also reveal whether the red blood cells are small and lacking in haemoglobin (iron deficiency) or larger than they should be (B12 or folate deficiency). The levels of iron (ferritin), B12 and folic acid can then be measured directly on another blood sample to confirm the cause of the anaemia.

Treatment consists of replacing the nutrients that are missing. If damage to the ileum means that vitamin B12 can no longer be absorbed, it must be given by injection for the rest of the patient's life, ordinarily 1mg of hydroxycobal-amin (B12) every three months. This certainly restores levels of haemoglobin and B12 to normal levels, but some patients find that fatigue recurs some weeks before their next injection is due, despite the normal blood tests. Some GPs will agree to give the injections more frequently to overcome this problem, which is still not fully understood. Some researchers believe that there is an 'active' form of B12 (transhydroxycobalamin) and that the level of this is more relevant when judging the amount of B12 replacement required.

Folic acid replacement is usually less of a problem. Damage to the small intestine has to be very severe indeed for simple supplements by mouth not to work very satisfactorily.

Iron supplements are often a problem in patients with IBD. It is usual to prescribe iron salts (such as ferrous sulphate or gluconate) but these often cause side-effects on the gut even in healthy patients, and these are much worse in those with IBD. I usually recommend therefore a liquid iron preparation, sodium iron edetate (Sytron). This can be started in a low dose of 10mls daily and built up to the maximum dose, which produces no ill-effects, but it is unusual for patients with IBD to be able to tolerate the full dose of 30mls daily.

Sometimes it is necessary to give iron by injection. Intramuscular injections may be painful and stain the overlying skin brownish-black. Intravenous iron has to be given in hospital, as it may lead to allergic reactions. Fortunately, recent preparations in which iron is linked to sucrose are less likely to have this effect.

Occasionally, especially in the presence of severe inflammation, blood transfusion may be necessary to correct anaemia, but its effects are not long-lasting.

Intestinal stricture: this is a narrowing of a portion of the bowel caused by inflammation, scarring or by cancer. The inflammation healing leads to formation of scar tissue, which has a tendency to contract. Such contraction may narrow the bowel and lead to slowing of intestinal flow or even complete obstruction.

Strictures tend to be more common in people with CD, although they are also reported in UC. The most common site for a stricture is in the small bowel, especially the terminal ileum. They may, however, arise in the large intestine particularly at anastamoses – that is to say, places where the bowel has been rejoined after a diseased portion has been removed at surgery. Common sites of large intestinal strictures include the rectum and transverse colon.

Symptoms of a stricture vary depending on its site, but usually include abdominal cramps, which become worse after eating. When the stricture becomes tight it may lead to constipation and even to nausea and vomiting. Sometimes acute intestinal obstruction may arise, where the flow of gut contents is blocked completely. This will cause acute abdominal pain and constipation followed shortly afterwards by abdominal distension, nausea and vomiting. In most cases such obstruction will settle spontaneously if the patient stops eating, and the upper gut is emptied by aspiration via a tube passed through the nose into the stomach (naso-gastric tube) and the patient is given intravenous fluids to prevent dehydration and loss of vital chemicals such as sodium and potassium. Sometimes, however, emergency surgery to relieve the blockage may be necessary.

If a stricture is suspected it can be confirmed by X-rays or endoscopy.

Some bowel cancers may present as strictures. However, strictures are usually not cancerous but full investigation may be necessary to confirm this including endoscopy and biopsies. The treatment of strictures will vary according to how narrow they are and whether they are produced by acute inflammation of the bowel wall or by scarring. If it is thought that the stricture is inflammatory, the standard anti-inflammatory treatment, such as diet or corticosteroids, may be sufficient to settle the inflammation sufficiently for the stricture to be relieved. If it is due to scarring these measures will not be adequate. A short stricture may be dilated at endoscopy. It is quite simple at colonoscopy to pass a balloon through a stricture to inflate it in order to stretch it. Likewise some small bowel strictures can be dilated at double-balloon enteroscopy.

Long fibrotic strictures and complex inflammatory strictures usually ultimately require to be removed at surgery. In the short term there may be relief from obstructive symptoms by taking a liquid feed (enteral diet) or in less severe cases by having a low-residue diet with no coarse fibre seeds and nuts.

Small intestinal bacterial overgrowth (SIBO): as we have seen, the small bowel in health contains very few bacteria. When strictures occur, however, the smooth flow of contents along the intestine is hampered, and under these conditions bacteria may be able to survive in the parts of the gut where flow is sluggish. Bacterial overgrowth may lead to diarrhoea and pain, and malabsorption of nutrients, which may cause weight loss. If SIBO is suspected, it may be confirmed by a glucose-hydrogen breath test (see page 78). The treatment in the short term is a course of suitable antibiotics, but it is better, if possible, to remove the stricture so that there is nowhere for bacteria to lodge. A final decision will depend on the nature and site of the stricture. If it is decided to continue with antibiotics, these are usually changed at intervals to prevent the bacteria becoming resistant to them.

Fistula: a fistula is an abnormal passage between two adjacent organs in the body. Fistulae are uncommon in ulcerative colitis. Because CD affects the whole wall of the gut with inflammation passing through from the inside of the bowel to the outside, it is possible for inflamed loops of gut to come into contact with other organs and for the inflammation to spread through into the adjacent organ. Thus fistulae may develop between one loop of bowel and another or between bowel and other structures such as the bladder, the skin and the vagina. Fistulae may occur after surgery, particularly if the wound has been infected and in these circumstances they may become long and tortuous and difficult to deal with.

Fistulae into the bladder cause urinary infections. Patients develop pain on passing urine and the urine may contain blood. Sometimes gas from the bowel may get into the bladder through a fistula leading to the passage of bubbles in the urine, a symptom known as pneumaturia. Such an infection is straightforwardly treated with antibiotics, but it is necessary to close the fistula if further infections are not to occur.

A fistula between the bowel and the skin may arise after surgery, and is also commonly seen around the anus when fistula tracks pass from the wall of the rectum and open out on to the skin surrounding the anus. These may start as a painful red lump, which later breaks down and discharges matter. Fistulae around the anus may give rise to recurrent abscesses if the fistula does not drain freely and becomes blocked. This can be prevented by putting a silk thread, called a seton, through the fistula to prevent it becoming obstructed. Some fistulae around the anus are dealt with quite simply by laying open the overlying skin and allowing the wound to heal. Unfortunately, many fistulae start in the rectum above the anal sphincter. Laying open such a fistula would lead to damage to the sphincter and possible incontinence. Surgery is therefore not appropriate in these cases.

Fistula healing can sometimes be achieved by the use of infliximab (see page 120).

Fistulae between loops of bowel may often be quite asymptomatic and cause little difficulty. Sometimes, however, they may lead to a short circuit so that a loop of bowel is bypassed and the absorption of nutrients reduced. This sort of fistula may sometimes respond to treatment with infliximab, but many will require surgery.

Anal problems in CD: approximately 10–15% of patients with CD present in the first instance with symptoms affecting the anus. In all, as many as a third of patients with CD will suffer peri-anal complications. They are much less frequent in UC.

The mildest of these may merely be **skin lesions** such as redness and soreness of the skin around the anus due to diarrhoea or drainage of faecal fluids. In CD it is quite common for **fleshy red anal skin tags** to form and indeed these are often a great help in making the diagnosis. They may look alarming and may bleed but they are not dangerous, and it is usually a mistake to excise them surgically, as the scar often fails to heal, leaving a very painful sore. Ulcers and abscesses just beneath the anal skin are also a feature of CD.

There may be **lesions of the anal canal** itself. These include fissures which are painful splits in its lining. More severe disease may lead to ulceration there and sometimes this can cause narrowing of the anal passage or an anal stenosis.

The anus can be investigated by MRI scanning (page 69), and, of course, local damage around the rectum can often be seen at endoscopy. However, endoscopy may sometimes be too painful in the presence of marked inflammation or fissure and the examination may therefore need to be performed under an anaesthetic in the operating theatre. Pain from anal lesions can often be relieved by the application of an anaesthetic cream such as Lignocaine just before the bowels are opened. This may not always be practical, particularly if there is frequent diarrhoea.

Anal fissures may be perpetuated by spasm of the anal sphincter muscle and this can be encouraged to relax, speeding up the healing of the fissure by applying glyceryl trinitrate cream to the anus twice daily. Unfortunately this cream will be absorbed into the bloodstream and may cause unpleasant headaches so it must be applied very sparingly. If glyceryl trinitrate alone is not successful in healing the fissure, it may be better to apply it by smearing it on an anal dilator. This is a smooth tapering probe that can easily be inserted partway into the rectum, serving both to dilate the sphincter and to get the cream further inside. Anal dilators, which come in various sizes, may also be used to treat an anal stenosis – a narrowing or a stricture of the anal canal.

Finally, persistent fissures may be treated surgically. A lateral sphincterotomy involves making a small cut, under general anaesthetic, in the anal sphincter. This takes away spasm in the sphincter and thus allows the fissure to heal, but may also weaken the muscle somewhat, so this operation is usually only performed in cases where other treatments have failed.

Antibiotics may be required to control infection and abscesses and in some cases of recurrent abscess formation, a long-term dose may be required to maintain anal health.

Nutrition may help the healing process. The exact diet recommended may vary from case to case but an increase in calories and protein may be of value as may be a reduction in the fibre content of the diet and vitamin and mineral supplements.

The healing process may also be helped by resting. Rest may also ease the pain of abscesses which may be under more pressure and therefore more painful on standing or walking.

Incontinence of faeces may arise because of an incompetent anal sphincter as a result of previous surgery, the passage of loose stools, increasing age or poor anal control. This is usually managed by the administration of bulking agents, particularly Celevac and Normacol together with an antidiarrhoeal agent such as loperamide. These agents tend to be more effective when used together. The formation of a plug made out of lavatory paper and inserted just inside the anus may prevent soiling of the underwear. Various-sized pads to wear inside underclothes are also commercially available.

Strict anal hygiene is very important. Diarrhoea and leakage from the anus may cause soreness and irritation. Plain moist tissue wipes are more gentle and less abrasive to the skin around the anus than ordinary lavatory paper. Frequent warm baths and showers, washing the anal area with a shower connection or the use of a bidet is very helpful and should be performed after a bowel movement. Following bathing, the anus should gently be dried either by patting the area with a soft towel or use a stream of warm air from a hairdryer. This is not only less painful, but it is more effective in keeping the skin dry, which is important in promoting healing and preventing secondary fungal infection.

Large and painful abscesses may require surgery and drainage as well as antibiotics. In general, surgery for perianal disease is rarely advised. This is not only due to the poor healing rate, which has already been mentioned, but also the risk of incontinence following surgery. Many studies show that the degree of rectal involvement in CD has an important influence on the success rate of surgery. The greater the inflammation the poorer the response.

Rectal strictures are often associated with long-standing disease and periodic dilatation may help. This may be continued manually by patients at home. Anal dilators can be provided in a range of sizes and when well lubricated, if necessary with local anaesthetic agents, may prove very effective.

Finally, in very severe cases, faecal diversion through a colostomy or ileostomy may be required. Sometimes diversion of the faecal stream away from the inflamed area may allow healing of peri-anal infection although, unfortunately, the relief may only be temporary and the disease may reoccur when the stoma is closed. However, if patients are suffering from chronic ill health and incontinence that leads to major inconveniences day to day, the option of faecal diversion may allow a much improved quality of life.

Recto-vaginal fistula: a recto-vaginal fistula is a passage between the rectum and the vagina allowing the passage of small amounts of waste from the rectum into the vagina. This may lead to an offensive discharge and possible infection. There may also be the passage of wind through the vagina.

Small fistulae producing minor symptoms may require no treatment. However, larger and more complex fistulae may require more vigorous action. This may involve making the stool firmer so that less is likely to pass into the vagina. This can be done by anti-diarrhoeal agents such as loperamide or by bulk laxatives such as Normacol and Celevac. Antibiotics may be necessary to reduce local infection and sometimes to prevent this occurring, a seton can be placed as stated above, allowing drainage to occur.

In some cases, vaginal douching is important to ensure that faecal fluid does not remain in the vagina. Flushing out the vagina with warm water will help to keep it clean. If you're unsure how to do this effectively, please ask your doctor or another health professional for guidance and advice.

Surgical repair of a recto-vaginal fistula is often difficult and many surgeons recommend a conservative approach. Its feasibility depends on a number of factors including the presence of active disease in the rectum, any associated infection and the degree of rectal involvement. Drug treatment such as immunosuppressants and corticosteroids will delay healing and make surgery more difficult and it may sometimes be necessary to do a temporary ileostomy to divert the faecal stream away from the rectum and vagina to allow a fistula to heal more satisfactorily.

This is a complex area that must be discussed in detail with your surgeon. Even in the best hands, recto-vaginal fistulae may return and many women choose to live with the problem rather than undergo complex surgery. The presence of such a fistula does not prevent the use of tampons at menstruation but these may be uncomfortable, in which case sanitary towels may be preferred.

Sexual intercourse will not make the fistula worse but may be uncomfortable. Due to the presence of faecal discharge, intercourse may seem inappropriate, but a condom may be used. Likewise there is no contraindication to using a diaphragm as most recto-vaginal fistulae are low down, that is, below the cap, which is therefore still an effective contraceptive.

Aphthous ulcers: CD can affect any part of the gastrointestinal tract and sometimes affects the mouth. Aphthous ulcers are small white superficial lesions with a red margin. They are usually around half a centimetre in diameter and can be single or multiple and occur anywhere in the mouth. Painful ulcers on the tongue and the lining of the mouth are, of course, very common in the general population and are quite separate from CD. They are, however, much more common in patients with CD and repeated crops of mouth ulcers with little respite should be an indication for further investigation.

Oral disease may be the first evidence of CD particularly in children and teenagers. This may cause disfiguration of the lips, which can be most distressing but which fortunately tends to resolve completely with time.

A condition known as orofacial granulomatosis is strongly linked with CD and may possibly be another form of it. It particularly affects the lips and gums. The ulcers produced by CD may be very painful.

However, all manifestations of CD respond well to diet (see chapter 5) which should be tried in an early stage in *all* patients suffering these difficulties. In the short term, oral ulcers may be eased by antibiotic suspensions, steroid ointments, antacid suspensions or when they are very painful, local anaesthetic gels.

Abscess: we have seen before (page 153) how CD, by causing inflammation of the whole bowel wall, may lead to fistulae. Such fistulae may open into adjacent organs or they may lead to the formation of an abscess. An abscess is most likely to develop when CD is chronically active and in particular if there is a degree of obstruction to the intestine. Long-term treatment with corticosteroids makes abscesses more likely. Often a communication between the bowel and the abscess can be demonstrated and the abscess may complicate previous surgery.

The majority of such abscesses are in the abdominal cavity, but they also occur in the pelvis and between the peritoneal cavity and the muscles of the back. This latter group may cause confusion by producing pain, which spreads to the hip or the knee rather than into the abdomen (psoas abscess).

As a basic principle, abscesses have to be drained. Antibiotics alone are insufficient to deal with them, although they may be very helpful to stabilise the situation before surgery or to prevent the spread of bacteria from the abscess into the blood (septicaemia). Nowadays, it's often possible to drain an abscess percutaneously, i.e. by passing a needle under X-ray control through the skin and, avoiding other abdominal organs, into the abscess so that the pus can be sucked out. It is still frequently necessary to drain abscesses by open surgery and it may be necessary at the same time to remove a loop of bowel, particularly if it's shown that this communicates with the abscess cavity or if there is a stricture.

Gallstones: these may affect as many as 10% of the population, but occur even more frequently in patients with CD. In one study in Birmingham 20% of CD patients had gallstones. This is because most gallstones form as a result of the formation of crystals of cholesterol in the bile. Cholesterol is kept in solution in the bile by the bile salts. If there is disease of the terminal ileum, or if this is removed surgically, the normal reabsorption of bile salts and their transfer back to the liver (see page 81) is interrupted. However, there is also a relationship with the number of operations patients have undergone and it is possible that disturbances to the flow of bile post-operatively may also be important.

Most people know that the gallbladder is situated in the upper right-hand side of the abdomen and expect gallbladder pain to be felt in that position. However, it's usually only when there is acute inflammation of the gallbladder (cholecystitis) that pain is felt there. More typically, biliary pain is felt in the centre of the upper abdomen and is worse after meals particularly when they are fatty. It spreads to the back and characteristically to the right shoulder and shoulder blade and is often associated with nausea and belching.

Such symptoms should always be further investigated.

Effects on the liver: blood from the intestine flows through the portal vein to the liver to be filtered and cleansed before it is released back into the circulatory system. It might be expected therefore that the liver would often be involved in cases of IBD.

Sometimes patients with IBD have abnormal liver function tests, but this may merely reflect inflammation elsewhere in the gut rather than any particular liver problem. However, it has been suggested that people with IBD are more susceptible to the damaging effects of alcohol upon the liver. It would be very surprising if IBD did not affect the liver and, in fact, biopsies with patients with apparently normal liver function show that as many as half of them have abnormal appearances. In many there is an increased amount of fat in the liver (steatosis) which probably reflects chronic inflammation and perhaps a degree of malnutrition which fortunately does not appear to progress to cirrhosis. Mild liver inflammation (hepatitis) is sometimes present.

The most important complication affecting the liver is primary sclerosing cholangitis.

Primary sclerosing cholangitis (PSC): this is much commoner in UC than in CD. At least 70% of patients with PSC have UC.

PSC slowly reduces the rate of flow of bile along the bile duct. This may result in jaundice, itching, pale stools and dark urine. In the presence of jaundice, it may be possible to relieve the blockage in the bile duct by dilating the gut with a balloon at endoscopy or by putting in a small plastic drainage tube known as a stent to keep the duct patent. PSC may also lead to cirrhosis of the liver. These are serious complications, but PSC may now be treated successfully by liver transplantation. Over 75% of patients transplanted for PSC are well ten years later. PSC is most commonly diagnosed by MRI (see page 69) although sometimes it may be necessary to perform an endoscopic retrograde cholangiopancreatograph (ERCP) to confirm the diagnosis and possibly to relieve strictures in the bile ducts.

In the short term the flow of bile may be improved by giving extra supplements of bile salts in the form of ursodeoxycholic acid. It's also important to try and keep the underlying IBD under close control. In a number of cases the bowel symptoms from patients with IBD and PSC are relatively minor and they seem to do well on 5-aminosalicylic acid alone. Other cases progress more rapidly and each has to be assessed on its own merit. Sometimes, PSC progresses even when a colectomy has been performed for UC.

Patients with PSC are at a substantially increased risk of developing cancer in the bile ducts (cholangiocarcinoma) and also at an increased risk of cancer of the large intestine, over and above that resulting from UC. This is discussed in more detail in chapter 9.

It should be stressed that sclerosing cholangitis is rare and the incidence in UC is no more than 1–4%.

Arthritis in IBD: patients with IBD are at increased risk of a number of joint conditions. It has been suggested that as many as 10–20% of patients may be affected.

The arthritis associated with IBD has been classified by researchers in Oxford into two types on a simple count as to whether fewer than five joints are affected (Type I) or more than five (Type II). Type I arthritis was seen in 3.6% of patients with UC and in 6% in CD, whereas Type II occurred in 2.5% of patients with UC and 4% of those with CD. Arthritis often produces persistent symptoms that may be independent of the activity of the IBD. The importance of IBD in causing arthritis can be deduced from one study in which leucocyte scans, to show gastrointestinal inflammation, were performed in patients with arthritis who had no gut symptoms. The scans were positive, showing gut inflammation in no less than 53%. Clearly the link between the bowel and the joints is close.

The joints most often affected in IBD are small- or medium-sized, such as the ankle, wrist, elbow and knee.

Sulphasalazine is often used to treat arthritis in IBD as it is effective against both inflammation in the joints as well as the gut. Non-steroidal anti-inflammatory drugs (NSAIDs) can also be used for the relief of pain and inflammation in joints, but these sometimes upset the gut in patients with IBD and so they are of less value. Controlling the gastrointestinal inflammation is often successful in reducing the arthritis.

Ankylosing spondylitis (AS): ankylosing spondylitis is a rheumatic disease affecting the spine and particularly the sacroiliac joint between the lower part of the vertebral column and the hip bone (sacroiliitis). It is 30 times more common in patients with UC than it is in the general population, but overall it is an infrequent disorder and the risk of developing it in IBD is small.

Following periods of inflammation as healing occurs, bone grows out from both sides of the vertebrae (bones of the spine) and may join them together, causing stiffness and immobility. When this is markedly developed, the appearances are of a 'bamboo spine'.

The cause of AS is unknown, but there are certain factors which may make one predisposed to the condition. The risk is increased if a first-degree relative also has IBD; there is a genetic tendency towards the disease. About 90% of patients with AS have inherited the gene for HLA-B27. However, when AS occurs together with IBD, HLA-B27 is only positive in about two-thirds of patients. Many members of the general population have an HLA-B27 gene but never develop the disease.

AS is a progressive disease and starts off with minimal effects such as low backache, which gradually gets worse over time. Other signs may be of stiffness, aches and pains in the neck, shoulder and hip and a sciatica-type pain felt down the back of the thigh. These may be mild and intermittent and cause little difficulty or more active when with the patient is tired, ill or has lost weight.

At the same time, other joints, particularly the hip, knee and ankle, may be affected.

The diagnosis is made by a straight X-ray of the spine on which the changes are usually clearly apparent.

This disease is progressive and incurable, but symptomatic relief is achievable and most sufferers can enjoy a full life. The aim of medical treatment is to relieve the pain and inflammation and to help the patient keep fit and healthy. Physiotherapy is very important and sulphasalazine and NSAIDs may also be very useful. Local heat and straightforward painkillers such as paracetamol may be very valuable. Posture is important. It should be the aim to keep the back straight at all times and avoid stooping over a desk at work or sitting in one position for too long without moving the back. Corsets and braces may make the condition worse as muscles that support the back may be weakened by immobility. A firm bed may provide more comfort in keeping the spine straight and if necessary a board can be inserted under the mattress to provide more support.

Sport and exercise may help; swimming allows good use of all muscles and joints without leading to weight-bearing injury.

Diet may help in AS. It has been suggested that a bacterium called *Klebsiella* has been isolated from the stools of patients with AS and may cross-react immunologically in some way with HLA-B27. It has been suggested that a low-carbohydrate diet may reduce the activity of this organism and help slow the progression of the disease, but this remains unproven.

Occasionally surgery may be carried out to provide movement in damaged hip joints. Rarely, surgery to the neck or back may be necessary to straighten the deformities. However, this is unusual and most cases will gradually burn out with patients being left with little more than a stiff back, which does not prevent general mobility. However, the importance of maintaining exercise and good posture cannot be overemphasised.

Osteoporosis: patients with IBD develop thin bones. There is still debate whether this is due to chronic inflammation in the gut or to the effects of corticosteroids, which are well known to promote osteoporosis. The problem is usually worse in patients with CD rather than UC. Mild thinning of the bones, or osteopaenia, occurs in about 50% of cases and the more severe osteoporosis in at least 10%. Both are more common in those who smoke, and there is evidence of a direct association between bone loss and IBD activity. However, this link may simply reflect increased corticosteroid usage in more active disease.

We performed a study in which bone densities were determined in patients with CD who had been treated predominately by corticosteroids, by diet or by non-steroidal drugs, with or without surgery. We compared the bone densities with those found in healthy people of the same ages. We found that although bone density was clearly reduced in those patients who had been treated with corticosteroids, the results in the other two groups were no different from our normal controls.

Some people believe that most bone is lost when corticosteroid treatment is first begun and that recurrent short courses may therefore be more damaging than long-term treatment.

Osteoporosis is important because sufferers are at a greater risk of a bone fracture. Fortunately, treatment is available. All patients who are started on corticosteroids should also receive generous supplements of calcium and vitamin D. A common prescription is Calcichew 2 tablets daily and if evidence exists of early bone loss, this should be increased to Calcichew – D_3 Forte. More severe cases are treated with chemicals known as biphosphonates, which increase the incorporation of calcium into bone. Using these drugs it is quite possible to reverse the progress of osteoporosis and even to increase bone density towards normal levels.

Kidney disease: kidney stones are more common in patients with IBD. These may be comprised of calcium oxalate or calcium urate. They are thought to be due to increased reabsorption of oxalate from the large bowel, particularly in patients who have had extensive small bowel surgery. The oxalate is excreted in the urine and may lead to stone formation.

The urate stones are less common and may be caused by dehydration. This is more likely to occur when there has been extensive small bowel surgery leading to loss of large amounts of fluid in the stools. It may not be sufficient merely to try drinking more liquids to overcome this; sometimes rehydration solutions containing glucose, sodium chloride and bicarbonate will be necessary (see chapter 8).

Kidney stones may cause blockage of the ureters and this may cause back pressure on the kidneys (hydronephrosis). Hydronephrosis may also develop particularly in the right kidney when there is chronic inflammation in the gut immediately overlying the kidney.

Kidney damage may result very occasionally in patients taking 5-ASA therapy and kidney function should be checked annually in these patients.

Eye problems: patients with IBD may develop inflammation in the eyes. This is more common in those who suffer from arthritis and in general is associated with active disease in the bowel. It appears to be commoner when the IBD affects the colon rather than the small intestine.

The commonest way in which the eyes may be affected is episcleritis. This causes burning or itching of the eye, which will also water, and occurs in 3–4% of patients. On examination the eye looks a little reddened as in conjunctivitis, but occasionally the inflammation is more severe with disturbances in vision or small ulcers developing. Treatment with steroid drops is not always required, but is usually very effective. As episcleritis is associated with increased activity of disease, getting the intestinal inflammation under control is always crucial.

A more severe eye disease is called iritis or uveitis. This presents with an acutely painful inflamed red eye and with disturbance of vision. There is a risk of permanent damage if prompt treatment is not initiated. If there is any doubt about the diagnosis, an ophthalmologist can confirm the inflammation by examination of the eye with a slit-lamp.

Treatment is usually with steroid eye drops together with drops to dilate the pupil. If the eye is very painful simple analgesics are usually effective. Again, it is important to bring gastrointestinal inflammation under control.

Skin problems: patients with IBD, especially young women, may develop red spots on the face – a condition known as rosacea, which usually responds well to steroid creams and sometimes antibiotics.

A more typical lesion which is usually a sign of active

CD is *erythema nodosum*. This produces painful raised dark red lesions, typically on the legs, especially the shins, and is commoner in relatively young patients. Although it may affect as many as 15% of patients with CD, only 2% of those with UC are affected. It usually implies a flare-up of inflammation of the gut and settles when that is adequately treated. Specific treatment for the skin is usually not required.

A much less common form of skin disease is *pyoderma gangrenosum*. This only affects about 2% of patients and is more common in long-standing disease, usually when there is inflammation in the bowel.

The *pyoderma gangrenosum* may respond to the treatment prescribed for the bowel disorder, but sometimes treatment dosages have to be increased considerably. Injection of steroids into the lesion or the application of potent steroid ointments beneath heavy dressing is also very valuable.

Sweet's syndrome is a very rare condition sometimes described in both UC and CD. This causes tender purple red nodules on the skin, usually on the arms, face or neck and usually responds to corticosteroids.

Thrombosis: a number of clotting abnormalities are present in the blood of patients with active IBD and this can increase the risk of their developing a DVT where blood clots occur in the veins of the legs and pelvis and which may sometimes break off to lodge in the pulmonary artery obstructing blood flow, which is known as a pulmonary embolus. Thrombosis may also occur in the artery supplying the gut and the brain.

In one Austrian study, the risk of such thrombo-embolic disease was nearly seven times greater in patients with IBD than in age- and sex-matched controls.

The risk of thrombosis is not such that specific treatment

is required for all patients with IBD; the standard treatment to bring inflammation under control is sufficient to reduce the risk of thrombosis occurring. Patients admitted to hospital, however, where immobility may increase the risk of thrombosis even further, should be given subcutaneous injections of low molecular weight heparins such as Enoxaparin, Tinzaparin and Dolteparin.

When patients with IBD do develop DVT, they should be treated in the standard way with heparin and then with oral anti-coagulant such as Warfarin. This is safe and will not normally lead to dangerous gastrointestinal bleeding, even though there may be ulceration in the gut.

Chest problems: UC appears to be more often complicated by respiratory problems than CD. Patients may develop dilatation and chronic infection of the air passages, a condition known as bronchiectasis. This usually progresses very slowly and responds well to treatment, whether with antibiotics or corticosteroids. CD is more likely to produce obstruction and granulomatous inflammation in the smaller air passages (bronchiolitis), again with slow progression and satisfactory response to standard treatments.

Deafness: there appears to be an increased likelihood of deafness in both UC and CD. One study suggests that as many as 10% of patients with IBD under the age of 50 can be demonstrated to have mild hearing impairment when this is carefully tested by audiometry. Any deafness in IBD patients should be reported immediately so that treatment can be instituted before permanent damage occurs.

Thus, although IBD is primarily an intestinal disease, it may lead to damage of many distant organs, which may require specific, separate treatments. However, it remains of prime importance that the inflammation in the gut is kept under control, as this will not only help the management of extraintestinal complications but will also ensure that new ones do not develop.

CHAPTER 8

Surgery in IBD

This is not a surgery textbook. It takes many years of arduous training to become a colo-rectal surgeon and there is no need for you to be burdened with all the knowledge that your surgeon requires. In this chapter I hope to let you understand the role of surgery in IBD better, to explain why it may become necessary, what procedures may be performed and what is likely to happen to you if you and your doctors agree that surgery is the best way forward.

The decision to undertake surgery will not be taken lightly by your medical team and nor should it be taken lightly by you. It's important that you feel at ease with your surgeon and able to talk with him freely. Many centres now have joint clinics for IBD patients where they are seen both by a physician and a surgeon and it may be that you have come to know the person who will do your operation quite well long before the final decision to operate is taken. This may make things easier, but even if you meet the surgeon for the first time just beforehand, do not be overawed. He owes a duty to you as his patient and you are perfectly entitled to ask him about anything you don't understand or which may be troubling you. It may help to write down a list of questions you would like to raise so that you don't forget them and regret it afterwards.

Remember, too, that surgery can only be performed if you sign a consent form that sets out what surgery is proposed and what its effects will be and that you have had the opportunity to discuss the matter and have any questions answered. Sometimes, in an emergency surgery, has to be done quickly, but there must still be time for you to understand very clearly what has been suggested and to make sure that you agree with it.

SURGERY IN UC

Surgical operations fall into two groups:

1. Emergency: performed at very short notice because an emergency has arisen.
2. Elective: performed after careful consideration at a time of the patient's and the doctor's choosing.

EMERGENCY SURGERY

It is not at all common for emergency surgery to be required in UC. There are four major reasons why it may be necessary:

❭ Acute severe disease which is not responding to medical treatment

❭ Acute uncontrollable bleeding from large intestine

❭ Toxic dilatation of colon (megacolon)

❭ Perforation

Acute UC which does not respond to medical treatment (see page 132) is a medical emergency. Patients with this problem will be admitted to hospital and monitored very carefully. Pulse and temperature will be taken every six hours and the stool frequency and consistency recorded daily. The presence of blood in the stool and any abdominal tenderness are important and the activity of the bowel may be checked by the doctors by listening to the bowel sounds with a stethoscope. Blood will be checked daily and a straight abdominal X-ray will be taken to see if there is any sign of dilatation of the large bowel. If these observations suggest that the patient is not responding, then elective surgery is usually recommended.

This is because toxic dilatation is a very dangerous condition in which the bowel distends so much that it is in danger of perforating. Toxic dilatation causes abdominal pain, nausea, vomiting, fever and dehydration. If a perforation does occur then some of the contents of the bowel will escape into the abdominal cavity and this leads to peritonitis, which can be life-threatening. Thus the development of a toxic colon is a clear indication for surgery.

Uncontrollable bleeding from the bowel is again uncommon. Bleeding from the mucosa is, of course, characteristic of UC and although it may lead to anaemia, it is rarely dangerous in itself. Sometimes, however, severe bleeding develops and this again is an indication for emergency colectomy.

ELECTIVE SURGERY

Elective colectomy is done for two main reasons. The most common is that medical treatment has been relatively unsuccessful so that the disease severely limits a patient's lifestyle. Despite continuing medication, symptoms may never really settle and there may be persistent complications affecting for example, the joints, the skin or the eye (see chapter 7). As with many long-term illnesses, general health can slowly become worse. Patients may feel too tired and wan to pursue a full range of activities, and anxieties about abdominal pains, diarrhoea and possible accidents may make them increasingly reluctant to leave the safety of home. Often patients themselves do not realise how much their lives have been limited by such chronic ill health and it's only after surgery, when the inflamed colon has been removed, that they realise how much better their health has become. Many patients who have surgery for this form of chronic UC say afterwards they wished they had had the operation earlier!

The second reason for elective surgery is the risk of progression to cancer. This is discussed in more detail in chapter 9. However, changes such as dysplasia in biopsies from the lining of the bowel may be an indication that it would be dangerous to leave the colon in place. Sometimes an early cancer may be revealed at colonoscopy. In this situation, clearly surgery is the best way forward.

SURGERY IN CD

The approach to surgery in CD is significantly different from that in UC. There are two reasons for this: the small bowel is likely to be involved rather than just the large; and because of the high rate of disease recurrence after surgical resection. It has been shown that 50% of patients with CD can expect to come to surgery at some time during their lives and of these another 50% will need a second operation within the next five to ten years.

Emergency surgery in CD is rarely needed for severe inflammation in the colon and for complications such as toxic megacolon, as these are very much less frequent in CD than they are in UC. Emergency surgery may, however, be needed to relieve intestinal obstruction caused by strictures, which may lead to perforation, or to deal with sepsis arising from intra-abdominal abscesses.

As in UC, elective surgery may be advised in cases of chronic disease that have responded poorly to medical treatment, although it is my impression that this is less common in CD than it is in UC. Fibrotic strictures causing repeated difficulties may require resection and, of course, some strictures in the small bowel may be malignant, although this is uncommon. Surgery may also be required to deal with fistulae (see page 153).

OPERATIONS CHOSEN

SURGERY FOR UC

Surgery for UC almost always means total removal of the large bowel. It may seem excessive to take away the whole colon when perhaps only the left side or even the sigmoid and rectum is inflamed, but experience has shown that attempts to remove the diseased part alone are fraught with difficulties. Almost inevitably the colon left behind becomes inflamed and the patient's symptoms continue relentlessly. Removing the whole colon, by contrast, produces a permanent cure of UC.

If the whole colon is removed, some form of procedure is necessary to allow the collection of the fluid that comes out of the small bowel. Initially an ileostomy is formed with a spout of small intestine, a stoma, that protrudes through the skin and is attached to a bag, into which the fluid can collect. This is a very safe and sure operation with good results. Sometimes there may be skin problems around the stoma, which may retract or be herniated, and sometimes there is intestinal obstruction. In 75% of cases, however, the stoma behaves perfectly well.

Nevertheless, it's not surprising that many patients are reluctant to undergo an operation that leaves them with a stoma and a bag. The modern alternative is to construct a pouch from loops of terminal ileum and to suture this to the anal canal, thus creating an internal pelvic pouch which discharges via the normal route. Afterwards, apart from the surgical abdominal scars, there is no trace that the large bowel has been removed. A trial performed in Leeds a few years ago has confirmed the value of ileo-anal pouches. Of 60 patients where surgery was performed, all were continent after one year and able to defer opening their bowels for at least 15 minutes. The median number of times a day that patients had their bowels opened was five and they rarely needed to get out of bed at night for this.

An ileo-anal pouch may be constructed in one, two or even three stages. It's generally wiser in a patient with severe colitis to have a simple colectomy and ileostomy at first, with the pouch created when the disease has gone into remission. There was a vogue for performing the whole procedure in one go in patients where it was performed electively, but nowadays many surgeons prefer a two-stage procedure. Initially a normal ileostomy is performed to allow the pouch surgery to heal. Later, when the pouch is ready to function, a second operation closes the ileostomy.

The main reason for pouches going wrong is infection around the anus or pelvis which may cause a great deal of discomfort and delay discharge from hospital, but which very rarely causes the loss of the pouch itself. Some patients are troubled by inflammation of the pouch known as pouchitis, which is discussed on page 187.

Nowadays, much abdominal surgery is 'keyhole' surgery – that is to say it is performed through a laparoscope inserted into the abdomen through the navel. This dramatically reduces the size of the incisions and allows the patient to make a much speedier recovery with less risk of complications. It is now possible to perform a colectomy and to construct a pouch with only a low transverse abdominal incision, which is not visible in a patient wearing bikini bottoms. Such elegant surgery will become increasingly available in the future.

SURGERY FOR CD

Surgery in CD is much more complex than that in UC. Even though the reoccurrence rate after surgery in CD is high, there is no need to recommend total colectomy in every case; the right side of the bowel or a segment can be removed in many cases, and if the disease does recur, managed by medical means.

This implies that there is usually less need to perform an ileostomy in CD, although sometimes this is unavoidable when patients have been taking large doses of prednisolone just prior to surgery. Prednisolone reduces the body's healing capacity and it may therefore be necessary to perform a temporary ileostomy to protect the joins between various loops of bowel when intestinal resections have been performed. When the whole of the large bowel is removed for CD, the subsequent relapse rate is very much less, being in the order of perhaps 15% rather than over 75%. This is further evidence of the importance of the bacteria of the colon in perpetuating CD.

Small bowel strictures can often be straightforwardly resected, with the healthy ends of the small bowel then being reconnected. However, removal of the small bowel may cause serious difficulties with the absorption of nutrients and fluid, and surgeons do their utmost to preserve the small bowel as far as possible.

This has led to the development of an operation called a stricturoplasty (see fig. 3). This is used to treat small bowel strictures. Instead of resecting the affected part of the bowel, the surgeon makes a longitudinal cut along the narrow piece of bowel (see fig. 3, B) and then stitches it up transversely at 90 degrees to the incision (fig. 3, D). This has the effect of widening the lumen of the bowel and is surprisingly effective. Even when the stricture is inflammatory, a stricturoplasty of this sort may allow that patch of CD to heal completely. Most surgeons will therefore choose to perform a stricturoplasty unless there is a very well-defined and relatively short section of affected small bowel, which can be resected without causing nutritional problems.

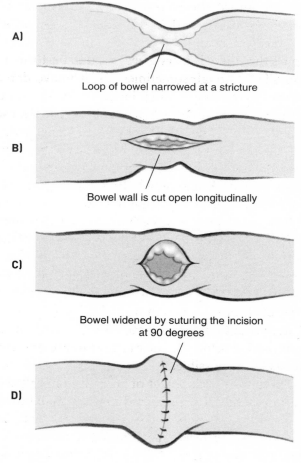

A) Loop of bowel narrowed at a stricture

B) Bowel wall is cut open longitudinally

C) Bowel widened by suturing the incision at 90 degrees

D)

Fig. 3: Stricturoplasty

The question of whether it's better to do segmental colectomy or remove the whole colon in CD remains somewhat controversial. One German study suggested that people treated by segmental colectomy did very well: after ten years of following these patients, only 1 in 10 needed to go on to a full colectomy. However, in a similar French study, as many as 50% of the patients went on to total colectomy within two years of the original operation. The presence of severe disease of the rectum and anus is an important factor influencing the outcome of surgery to the colon in CD. The best way forward for an individual patient will be a matter of careful discussion between the patient, the surgeon and the physician.

It is generally considered unwise to perform an ileo-anal pouch in CD. As the pouch is constructed from the small bowel, it may become the site of active CD with disastrous consequences, including complex fistulae and inflammation necessitating removal of the pouch itself. In one set of figures from the Mayo clinic in the USA, the overall failure rate was as high as 45%.

A number of factors have been discovered to be important in the risk of relapse after surgery for CD. Smoking in particular increases relapse rates. Although all patients with CD should *stop* smoking completely, certainly they should not smoke in the period immediately before and after surgery.

Attempts to reduce the risk rate by medication have not, to date, been of great success. My own current practice is to recommend that all patients with CD undergoing surgery, post-operatively follow a LOFFLEX (Low Fibre, Fat limited, Exclusion) diet; for more details see pages 93, 97). During this they can search for any possible food intolerances. A number of my patients have done very well following this route, but it has yet to be formally tested in a controlled trial.

GOING INTO HOSPITAL FOR SURGERY

Before you are admitted to hospital for an operation you will receive written information about what to bring in, such as clothing and toiletries and medication, etc. You may have to go into the ward the day before the operation in order to clear faeces out of the bowel by taking a bowel cleanser such as Picolax or Citromag. You will also have your general health checked by the house surgeon, who will look for any signs of problems that might mean that the surgery will need to be postponed. Blood pressure, pulse and temperature will be recorded so there is a base line which values can be compared to after the operation.

If an ileostomy is to be performed, the stoma care nurse will come and see you. She will give you preliminary details and discuss with you the ideal position for the stoma and mark it on your skin so that the surgeon can see where to put it. You will also be asked to sign a consent form for surgery. You are able to change your mind about this right up until the last moment, but obviously if you back out just before the operation, you will have deprived someone else of the chance of using that slot! The anaesthetist will come and visit you to check that you are fit for an anaesthetic and explain how it will be administered and talk you through post-operative pain relief. You will be asked not to eat or drink for several hours before the operation so that your stomach is empty and there is less risk of inhaling stomach contents under the anaesthetic. Further blood may be taken to make sure that you are not anaemic and to cross-match any blood that might be needed for transfusion.

After the operation you will probably wake up in the recovery room in the care of the nurses who will check your condition carefully until you are able to move back to the ward. In this early stage you will find that there are a number of tubes going into various parts of your body to give you fluids and medication or to drain urine and wounds. The anaesthetist may have provided 'patient-controlled analgesia'. This is an automatic pump with a lock on it to prevent overdose, which you can activate yourself when you feel discomfort. It may allow painkilling drugs to be pumped either into a vein or sometimes into the back by means of an 'epidural' – a fine needle placed in the spinal canal.

At first, to allow your gut to recover, you will not be able to eat, but after a few hours, you will be allowed to start drinking water and if this passes satisfactorily down the gut, food will gradually be reintroduced. At the beginning this will be soft and easily digestible. If you have CD you may be advised to start with some liquid enteral feeding or the LOFFLEX diet.

As your gut recovers, the various tubes will be removed and you will start taking painkillers by mouth. You will go on having subcutaneous injections of anti-coagulants to prevent blood clots forming in your legs and you will be encouraged to get out of bed to walk about as soon as you can as this also reduces the risk of a thrombosis.

If you have an ileostomy the stoma care nurse will come and show you how to look after it. This is discussed in more detail on page 183.

Most patients who undergo a colectomy are in hospital for 10–14 days, slightly longer if there are complications. During this time you will almost certainly feel tired and low. This is natural after such a major operation and you will find that as your health picks up, it rapidly clears. Sometimes depression occurs after surgery and, if so, you should discuss this with your doctor who will be able to help you overcome it.

When you get home you will have to stay off work for at least two months. At first your energy levels will be low and you will have to avoid heavy work such as lifting, making the bed and other household duties until the wounds have healed. Convalescence usually takes about two months but the time taken will obviously vary according to the extent of the surgery you have had and the state of your health beforehand. You may not be able to drive for several weeks and should not go back to work until you are fully recovered.

Gentle exercise is very helpful to speed recovery. Try taking a short walk or your doctor may suggest an exercise plan. If you have a stoma, then at this stage the stoma nurse will be invaluable in helping you to get used to managing it and dealing with any problems you may encounter. You should not be afraid to go and ask the medical team whenever you have difficulties.

ILEOSTOMY

After food has passed along the small intestine mixed with digestive juices and the nutrients absorbed, it is very liquid. One of the functions of the colon is to absorb water from the fluid entering the caecum from the ileum to produce normally formed stools. If the small bowel were to be connected directly to the anus, the patient would suffer permanent diarrhoea.

Therefore, if the whole colon has been removed, it's necessary to collect the stools in a different way. The ileostomy was developed by Professor Brooke, a surgeon at St George's Hospital in London, and many thousands of patients have reason to be very grateful for his skill. The end of the small intestine is brought through an opening in the abdominal wall called a stoma and the liquid is collected in a leak-proof bag that is attached to the abdominal skin.

Temporary ileostomies may sometimes be created to allow surgical procedures further down the bowel to heal more easily, but if the large bowel has been removed and there is no plan to construct a pouch, then the ileostomy will be permanent.

The stoma nurse will have discussed with you, before the operation, where the ileostomy should be placed. It is usually on the lower right-hand side of the abdomen overlying the end of the small intestine. The position is important. You must be able to see the stoma easily and it must be accessible whether you are sitting, lying or standing. It should not get in the way of your usual clothing, such as belts, and it must avoid scars and abdominal creases.

Because the intestinal secretions contain many irritant enzymes, it's important that the stoma protrudes several centimetres above the skin. It therefore looks like a moist pink spout. Although it looks quite delicate, it has no sensory nerve endings and therefore there is no feeling in the ileostomy. It can be handled without discomfort or causing harm, but it is of course necessary to keep it clean and to wash your hands before and after touching it.

When it's first created the ileostomy appears bigger and it will later shrink back a little. For a few days nothing comes out of it and then semi-liquid matter appears. Although it passes through the abdominal wall, there is no sphincter muscle in an ileostomy and it's not possible to control the passage of fluid voluntarily from the bowel into the ileostomy bag.

The stoma nurse will initially fit a bag and empty it when it is full. However, as you recover from your operation, the nurses will teach you how to do this for yourself. The ileostomy bag fits round the spout of the ileostomy and is attached to the skin. When the bag becomes full, it's emptied into the lavatory without detaching it from the ring around the base of the stoma. This means that the bag is reusable for several days before it needs to be replaced.

Several different companies make ileostomy bags. It is very important to make sure that the ring is the right size so that it fits snugly over the stoma and there are no leaks. Most bags have a filter to release excess gas to eliminate smell.

With the help and support of the stoma care nurses you will soon get used to living with your ileostomy. It will be necessary to pay some attention to your food. The fluid coming in to the bag is usually semi-liquid, but this may vary according to your diet. It is sensible to try and avoid excessive gas. One might believe that because the large bowel has been removed, fermentation of food residues would cease. However, the lower end of the small bowel becomes colonised with bacteria when an ileostomy is created and therefore fibrous foods such as peas, beans and brassicas may lead to excessive gas formation, which is best avoided. Fizzy drinks and onions may have a similar effect. Likewise it's possible to have an obstruction near the opening of the stoma caused by indigestible foods such as sweetcorn, nuts and celery. However, no specific diet is necessary and you will soon learn which things suit you best. As ileostomy fluid is more liquid than normal faeces, it does mean that you need to drink more fluid in order to make up for the ileostomy losses. Take care not to become dehydrated. If you would like more information, are worried or have any problems in this area, have a chat with one of the hospital dietitians.

The ileostomy spout may sometimes cause a little difficulty either by retracting back into the abdomen so that it becomes difficult to attach the bag or prolapsing out, which may also be awkward. In some cases it is necessary to have a further operation to get it back into the right position.

Nevertheless, most people find they can lead a normal life with an ileostomy and the majority are just delighted to feel so much better when they no longer suffer the symptoms of UC which is responding poorly to medical treatment. The ileostomy need not stop vigorous exercise, although there may be difficulties with contact sports such as rugby or football.

It's perfectly possible to swim when you have a stoma. Special swim-sportswear is available to conceal appliances but are not generally needed as most swimsuits and trunks are suitable. Special activity pouches are obtainable which are small enough to be undetectable under swimwear. Stoma protectors are also available which can be worn over the stoma and adhesive tape may be applied to the appliance for extra security in case you are anxious about leakage.

ILEO-ANAL POUCH

If an internal pouch has been constructed, you may need to go back for a second operation three or four months later to complete the process. This will not happen until you are fully recovered from the first operation.

Although a patient with an internal pouch is able to go to the lavatory in the usual way, it does not function exactly as a normal bowel. In the first place, the pouch contents are more liquid than stools in the large intestine as the drying effect of the large bowel has been removed. Secondly the sphincter muscles that control the anus may not always be strong enough to control some leakage, particularly in bed at night. Pelvic floor exercises should be practised (your doctor can tell you how to do this) and until the muscles become stronger, it may be necessary to wear a pad to protect your clothing. It is common to need to empty the pouch between four and seven times a day and night-time incontinence may cause difficulty for a small proportion of people. At first problems with wind, discomfort and leakages may cause difficulties, but, with practice, these matters are soon overcome and most patients find that life with their internal pouch is vastly superior.

POUCHITIS

One complication that may occur is of pouchitis. In this condition there is inflammation of the pouch itself. This seems to be related to changes in the bacteria that live inside the pouch. It is much more common in people who have pouches constructed because they suffer from UC than in people who have pouches because they are at great risk, for genetic reasons, of developing colon cancer.

Although the small bowel is normally sterile, when the pouch is formed, it becomes recolonised with bacteria, which are very similar to those in the original colon. There may be an increased number of oxygen-loving bacteria and of clostridia – both organisms that are known to cause problems in patients with IBS.

Pouchitis leads to diarrhoea and sometimes bleeding from the anus. The diagnosis can be confirmed by a sigmoidoscopy and biopsy in the clinic. It must be distinguished from 'cuffitis' – persisting inflammation in the very narrow cuff of rectal tissue left after surgery at the site of the anastomosis with the anus.

Although it may be very irritating, it is rarely dangerous and fewer than 5% of pouches have to be removed again because of pouchitis. The standard treatment is antibiotics – usually metronidazole or ciprofloxacin. If these are insufficient, corticosteroids may be helpful. I have found that a

LOFFLEX diet is of great value in many stubborn cases but antibiotics must always be tried first.

There is now some success in treating pouchitis with probiotics (page 228), and a course of antibiotics followed immediately by a course of probiotic mixture such as VSL-#3, which contains eight different healthy bacterial species, may be very valuable, not only in treating established pouchitis, but also in preventing it.

CROHN'S DISEASE – PROBLEMS AFTER SURGERY

Colectomy cures UC. Unfortunately, surgery does not cure CD. The main problem after surgery therefore must be relapse. Because this is so frequent there is considerable discussion among medical experts about the best way to try and prevent relapse in patients that have undergone surgery. Corticosteroids appear to be of little value and 5-ASA medications are usually disappointing. One thing that certainly does make a difference is smoking. If you have not already stopped smoking now is the time to do it (see chapter 9).

I also encourage my patients, who have had surgery to go on to perform dietary studies (see chapter 5). Often the reason for failure of diet is the presence of strictures in the bowel. When the stricture has gone, the bowel bacteria no longer have a foothold on which they can persist and although no formal controlled trial of diet after surgery has yet been performed, the benefits to many of my patients have been clear. Indeed, nowadays, I suggest to many of my patients with difficult strictures that these are dealt with before their dietary studies begin.

Although medical opinion currently is against the construction of ileo-anal pouches in CD because of the risk of the pouch itself becoming involved, nevertheless from time to time this surgery does take place. Sometimes this leads to problems, such as abscesses or fistulae that can only be dealt with by further surgery. CD in ileo-anal pouches, however, in my experience responds satisfactorily to dietary treatment and this should be the first approach if at all possible.

SHORT-BOWEL SYNDROME

The small bowel, as we have seen, is crucial for the digestion of food and the absorption of nutrients. Some parts of the bowel, such as the ileum, are specifically adapted to absorb items that cannot be taken up elsewhere. Vitamin B12 can be absorbed virtually throughout the ileum and resection of a few centimetres does not always lead to vitamin B12 deficiency. However, it's sensible to check B12 absorption post-operatively if this is possible. Bile salts, however, are absorbed specifically in the terminal ileum and quite a small resection in this area may lead to bile salt malabsorption and diarrhoea (see page 81).

Major resections of small bowel leaving less than 200cm may cause difficulties, which are known as 'short-bowel syndrome', where there is excessive loss of water and minerals, which may lead to malnutrition. Because surgeons are very aware of this possibility, short-bowel syndrome is unusual. The patient may be aware of diarrhoea or excessive fluid loss through a stoma and this inevitably leads to thirst. Fluids lost from the small bowel, however, contain a lot of sodium as well as water and the fluids available for thirsty patients don't usually contain much salt. Trying to replace liquid by drinking water alone stimulates more small-bowel secretion with the loss of yet more sodium, making matters worse.

For this reason, rehydration solutions have been developed which contain salt, sugar and sodium bicarbonate. These are much better for replacing fluid loss in this situation than are water or soft drinks alone.

Sometimes, because of short-bowel syndrome, it is necessary to feed the patient intravenously. This is known as total parenteral nutrition (TPN). Because the very rich solutions required to maintain nutrition in this way irritate the lining of veins and lead to thrombosis and inflammation, it's necessary to put the cannula involved into a large vein near the heart. These veins will not develop such problems, but having a cannula in such a central position carries other risks, in particular infection. There are also risks of haemorrhage or puncturing a vital organ when the cannula is positioned. For these reasons TPN is supervised by an expert team of specially trained nurses, dietitians and pharmacists, and it is necessary to look after the cannula extremely carefully.

The aim of TPN is to maintain a patient's nutrition by intravenous feeding while measures are taken to improve the capacity of the short small intestine to absorb nutrients. Apart from rehydration solutions, the patient is given drugs that reduce acid secretion and nutrition is supplemented with liquid feeds that are often pre-digested so they are more rapidly absorbed high in the small intestine.

Full discussion of such complex matters is beyond the scope of this book, but patients who develop this problem will find that they receive vigorous encouragement and support from the nutrition team in their own hospital.

Sometimes patients with a short gut have to be maintained indefinitely on TPN. Very rarely, technical problems with intravenous feeding mean that such patients must be considered for small bowel transplantation, which is a highly specialised procedure carried out in a small number of national specialist centres.

Surgery is frequently a highly successful treatment for IBD. When the condition was first described it was usually the only effective treatment. Nowadays, many other options are available but surgery remains an excellent choice for many longstanding and complicated cases. If your medical advisors suggest surgery, by all means clarify with them what other alternatives may be available, but remember that frequently it produces a dramatic improvement in a patient's health.

CHAPTER 9

Living with IBD

PREVENTING RELAPSE

When you have completed the initial treatment for your IBD
and are once again feeling well and optimistic you will naturally wish to stay that way. Both UC and CD are described
in the literature as diseases of relapse and remission, and it
is likely that some flare-ups may happen from time to time.
Nevertheless, you want to keep these down to the bare
minimum to avoid interference with your everyday life and,
of course, because the longer the disease is in remission, the
better is its chance of burning itself out completely.

The following tips may help to keep you well:

> ❯ If you are on a diet for CD, obviously you have to
> keep to that diet. There is a temptation to believe
> that if you feel well, there is no need to keep to the
> diet any longer. This is a trap and a delusion. If you
> eat foods that have been shown to upset you, you
> will eventually inevitably relapse. There are
> difficulties here in that sometimes you may find
> that you can eat an offending food once and
> discover that it causes very little in the way of
> symptoms. It's temping to believe that its effects
> may have passed off and go on eating it regularly.
> This is particularly true of foods made from flour
> such as sandwiches and biscuits, which are perhaps
> the most irritating to have to avoid.

❱ Unfortunately, when you have been well for some time, it may take several days or even weeks before foods start to upset you again. The offending bacteria have been suppressed by your diet. When you start to eat the dangerous foods, their numbers start to increase and it may be a little while before they are present in high enough concentration for the disease to be triggered off once more. It's usually at least five years (see chapter 5) before it's safe to go back to normal eating.

❱ Sometimes it may be difficult to avoid eating a forbidden food. At a wedding, for instance, food choices may be limited. Do let other people know which foods upset you. Restaurants are increasingly providing special menus. However, sometimes when you tell the waiter there are certain foods you have to avoid, the artistic chef may not be able to resist the temptation to add something (just proving his culinary skills!). Do not be embarrassed to demand exactly what you want. You are paying the bill and must be able to have the food that suits you!

❱ If you have UC, it's similarly important that you continue taking the medication as prescribed by your doctor or IBD nurse. Do not stop these medications because you feel well. If you do, you will relapse. The length of time for which it's necessary to continue medication in UC is difficult to gauge. There is no reliable way of knowing when the condition is so well controlled that it's possible to stop treatment or when stopping the medication will simply allow a relapse. I advise my patients with UC to continue until they have been completely asymptomatic for

three years before risking tailing off their
treatment.

❭ As soon as symptoms begin you should always seek
prompt advice or treatment in order to try and nip
the problem in the bud. This means that you must
always have an adequate supply of medications
available, particularly when you are travelling
away from home and out of easy contact from
your general practitioner. It's a good idea to keep a
small stock of medication available for
emergencies. If you have CD, a few cartons of
elemental diet in the cupboard may enable you to
settle down an early relapse in a couple of days
before serious problems arise. Likewise, a small
stock of enemas may be helpful to a patient with
UC, to start as soon as symptoms such as blood or
mucus in the stools arise. Enemas, of course, are
really only adequate for disease of the left-hand
side of the bowel, but you should not go on to oral
steroids or immunosuppressants without
instruction from your doctor.

❭ Remember that if you do have a sudden bout of
diarrhoea, this may not necessarily mean a relapse
of your IBD. Many people who have never heard of
IBD get bouts of diarrhoea if they have food
poisoning or dietary excesses. This may happen to
you as well. Gastroenteritis is a potent cause of
relapse of IBD, however, so if you do have
diarrhoea that lasts more than 24 hours, you
should arrange for a stool sample to be sent by
your doctor for culture to see if there is an infection
present. Your IBD nurse may well be able to help
you with this.

❭ It obviously also makes sense to avoid situations where gut infections are common. This includes travelling to countries which have poor sanitation or which are hot so that there is an abundance of flies. I usually advise my patients who wish to go on holiday abroad to choose Northern Europe or the USA. It's obviously important to maintain high standards of hygiene in preparing and cooking your own food (see page 208) and you would be well advised to avoid eating establishments which look to be casually maintained. However, it cannot be denied that it is possible to pick up food poisoning in the most salubrious environments. See also page 214 for further details.

❭ Some people with UC find that there are foods that trigger symptoms. Such foods should, of course, be avoided even though they represent only a minor part of the management of the condition.

❭ The link between stress and IBD is poorly understood (see page 42). Nevertheless, many people report relapses after stressful periods in their lives. It's important that you get adequate rest and sleep. This doesn't mean no partying, but balance late nights out with early nights at home. Make time in your life to follow hobbies and pursuits that you enjoy. If you can, take time to practise relaxation at certain periods every day. I believe that one of the most important effects of stress on the gut is rapid, shallow breathing – over-breathing – which leads to air swallowing, which in turn supplies oxygen to the gut bacteria. It's a good idea to take time to practise slow diaphragmatic breathing and relaxation. This technique is described in detail in another book I have written

(*Irritable Bowel Solutions*, Vermilion, 2007). In any case try not to bottle up worries or concerns, but discuss them with someone who may be able to help.

❱ Avoid constipation. Flares of left-sided colitis are frequently triggered by constipation further up the large bowel on its right side. The prevention of constipation is discussed on pages 145–147, 224.

❱ Avoid taking non-steroidal anti-inflammatory drugs (NSAIDs). A list of these is given in the table on page 41. They reduce the level of key defence hormones in the gut called prostaglandins. If you need to take a painkiller, try soluble paracetamol instead.

❱ Keep fit with regular exercise and eat a healthy balanced diet with vitamin and mineral supplements as necessary. Build up your bodily strength to reduce the risk of osteoporosis. Regular exercise is good for relieving stress and promotes relaxation and healthy sleep.

WHEN TO SEEK FURTHER TREATMENT

You should immediately see your doctor or phone your IBD nurse if you suffer any of the following problems:

✓ Severe abdominal pain or persistent painful swelling of the abdomen

✓ Vomiting for more than 24 hours

✓ Diarrhoea not responding to your usual IBD medication

✓ Bleeding from the back passage

✓ Weight loss

✓ Persistent tiredness or malaise (general feeling of being unwell)

✓ A change in bowel habit – e.g. diarrhoea to constipation or vice versa

✓ Side-effects or any unusual reactions to your medication as highlighted in the info sheets supplied with them

COMMON INFECTIONS

Compared to the complexities of IBD, everyday illnesses such as the common cold, sore throats and flu may seem trivial. However, such relatively minor problems should not be ignored as they may make the overall condition worse.

Colds and flu: these tend to strike when you are feeling low. Poor absorption or a lack of dietary intake of certain vitamins may increase vulnerability to such infections. If a cold persists for more than a few days without improving, you should let your GP know, especially if you are on medication. Some drugs depress the immune systems and, for example, the number of white cells in the blood may have become too low.

Treatments for colds and flu should include rest, so that you can conserve energy to allow the body to fight the infection. This is even more important if the CD or UC is active. You should also take plenty of fluids as the body can become dehydrated. Try to drink about three litres of liquid a day, especially if you have diarrhoea as a result of your IBD. Some people believe that high doses of vitamin C

(500mg–1g three times per day) may be helpful. Stores of vitamin C may certainly be low in patients with CD.

Sore throats: if you develop a sore throat you must contact your GP immediately if you are taking any of the following medications:

> Corticosteroids (prednisolone)

> Azathioprine (Imuran)

> Methotrexate

> Sulphasalazine

> Mesalazine (Pentasa, Asacol, Dipentum)

These drugs affect the immune system and you may need a blood test. If all is well simple remedies such as lozenges or gargles may help relieve the symptoms. Antibiotics are rarely necessary for a sore throat.

Vomiting: this may cause particular difficulties in patients with IBD because it may arise from an obstruction in the bowel. If so, it's usually associated with abdominal pain, tenderness and constipation. Vomiting of any sort may mean that you are not able to absorb your medications properly. If you are on corticosteroids this could be dangerous, as these must never be suddenly stopped without medical advice.

If vomiting continues for more than 24 hours you should always seek help from your doctor. Sometimes it's necessary to give fluids intravenously to prevent dehydration and patients on corticosteroids may need to have them injected.

Diarrhoea: despite taking the usual precautions to prevent gastroenteritis, this may occasionally occur. If so, you should treat it by replacing lost fluids: oral rehydration solutions such as Dioralyte are better than plain water. If these are not available a pint of boiled water with a teaspoon of salt and tablespoon of sugar added will serve very well. It is important to rest, and if the diarrhoea persists for more than 48 hours you should seek medical help. It's not advisable to take anti-diarrhoeals such as codeine or loperamide to stop diarrhoea as they may mask the potential cause and can lead to complications such as toxic megacolon (see page 128).

Urinary infection: these cause pain on passing urine (dysuria), increased frequency, pain in the back or side, malaise and fever. Blood may be visible in the urine. Although urine infections are not unusual, particularly in women, they may be a sign of a serious complication of IBD such as a fistula between the bowel and the bladder or stones in the urinary tract. In either case, prompt diagnosis and treatment is necessary and you should consult your GP without delay.

Toothache: strong analgesics will obviously help here. Unfortunately, some of the best come under the heading of NSAIDs, which, as we have said, are not recommended for IBD. Try simple analgesics such as soluble paracetamol or co-dydramol and arrange to see your dentist at an early stage to sort out the underlying problem.

Backache: simple backache can usually be resolved by painkillers and rest. Again, try to avoid NSAIDs. If the backache persists, despite these measures, consult your GP as it could be a complication of IBD such as sacroiliitis (see pages 53, 164).

IBD AND CANCER

There is undoubtedly an increased risk of cancer of the colon or small intestine in IBD. The good news, however, is that over 90% of patients will never develop it and even if you fall into one of the groups which are at increased risk, it is usually possible to detect the problem before serious damage is caused.

In UC there is an increased risk of colon cancer. It has been said that after 20 years of UC, 5–20% of patients will develop colorectal cancer, after 25 years perhaps 15% and after 35 years, up to 30%. Genetic factors may also be important, so a family history of colon cancer may again increase the risk.

The risk in UC depends on the extent of bowel inflammation. In proctitis and left-sided colitis, the risk of cancer is no greater than that of the general population. This does not mean that patients with proctitis and left-sided colitis cannot develop cancer, just that they are not at increased risk. People with pancolitis *are* at an increased risk. Attempts to quantify this risk are beset by all sorts of analytical difficulties. It's clear, however, that those patients in most danger are those with extensive long-standing, unresected colonic disease. This is true of both CD and UC.

The risk of developing bowel cancer is particularly high in patients with primary sclerosing cholangitis (PSC). These patients must be screened very carefully more frequently than those with uncomplicated UC (see page 162).

In patients with CD the risk of cancer of the large bowel is the same as that in patients with UC who have a similar extent of disease. The actual incidence is uncertain. Despite the increased risk of colon cancer in CD, fairly few cases are seen because it used to be very common to remove the colon in patients with CD who had responded poorly to medical treatment. This obviously prevents colon cancer from ever developing

Cancer in the small bowel is always rare. There is no increased risk of small bowel cancer in UC, but cancer is more likely to develop in the small intestine in patients with CD. The risk has been estimated at about six times that of the general population. Because of the extreme rarity of small bowel cancer in the general population, this means that the risk in CD is still small.

This may sound alarming. However, there is now evidence that keeping inflammation under control much reduces cancer risk. Taking regular treatment with 5-ASA may protect IBD patients against cancer, and nowadays most patients who have IBD for more than ten years are put into screening programmes for colonoscopies at regular intervals. There is no generally agreed programme for this and the frequency of examination varies from hospital to hospital. A typical approach is to recommend a colonoscopy every two to three years for people with UC extending from the anus to beyond the splenic flexure, which has been present for more than 10 years. After 15 years or, if abnormalities are discovered, the frequency of colonoscopy is increased.

At these colonoscopies, biopsies are taken to see if a change known as 'dysplasia' is present. This is a subtle change that indicates that a progression towards cancer may have started; it is not cancer itself. Dysplasia may be divided into low-grade changes, which are usually an indication for more regular screening, or high grade. When high grade is present, this usually means that cancer is likely to develop very shortly and most patients would be advised to have their colon removed. When dysplasia is associated with visible lesions in the bowel (DALM) it is of greater significance. Many colonoscopists now spray the lining of the colon with a blue dye to enable such lesions to be more easily visualised as they are the best place to take biopsies.

The small bowel, unlike the colon, is not easily accessible to screening techniques. It is sensible to be aware of the symptoms that may be occur. Cancers of the small bowel tend to occur in areas affected by underlying inflammation. Most occur in the terminal ileum and lead to further narrowing and obstruction. First they may produce an increase in abdominal pain, constipation and vomiting. Later on, there is a general deterioration in health with weight loss and fatigue.

Cancer in the large bowel may again cause increasing abdominal or peri-anal pain together with a change in bowel habit. This can be either constipation or diarrhoea. Often there will be blood in the motions.

In patients with large bowel cancer associated with IBD, it is wise to recommend removing the whole colon. Although it might be tempting just to do a segmental resection and to try rejoining the bowel again afterwards, the risk of further cancers developing is high, and removing the colon takes away all such risk. Cancers sometimes develop around the anus and rectum in patients with peri-anal disease, and in these cases, it will be necessary to do a colectomy and ileostomy as the anus is too damaged to be able to form an internal pouch.

Small bowel cancers can normally be dealt with by removing the lesion with any surrounding tissue that has been damaged by the inflammation and rejoining the ends of the healthy bowel. It is most unusual for further small bowel tumours to develop.

It's important not to be too frightened about the possible risks of cancer in IBD. Certainly the problem is there, but the means are available to handle it successfully. Some gastroenterologists recommend prophylactic colectomy – the removal of the large bowel without the development of dysplasia or any other lesions. This is certainly worth considering in people with long-standing disease that is not adequately controlled because surgery in these cases can lead to a most welcome improvement in general health and happiness and can at the same time remove the anxiety about the possible development of cancer. If you feel that you may be in this group, you should discuss the matter with your doctor.

A further factor that will reduce the risk of developing cancer in the years ahead is the development of new tests for its early diagnosis. For instance, groups are investigating the value of searching for genetic material (DNA) in the faeces or in colonic biopsies. Others are looking for metabolites in the body, which could be linked to the development of cancer. Immunological staining of biopsies may prove more sensitive and molecular biology is throwing up possible tumour markers, which may again enable earlier diagnosis to be achieved.

SMOKING AND IBD

CD patients who smoke have more serious complications, need more steroids and immunosuppressants and are more likely to require surgery than those who do not. It makes complete sense to GIVE UP.

The difficulty is of knowing how to do so. Many people – including some doctors – simply think it's just a matter of willpower. Sadly, willpower alone is rarely enough. Fewer than 1 person in 10 manages to give up smoking that way.

Our growing knowledge of the severe damage smoking causes to health has led to careful analysis being performed of the best ways to break the habit. Sadly, just being advised to stop smoking by a doctor or nurse has very little effect, even when the patient knows that smoking may be a factor causing the disease from which they are suffering. Nor does reading about the matter help very much. Hopefully, reading this book will have made you realise how important it is to stop smoking, but you are going to need much more help to do this!

Support is needed and results are better if this is provided, face to face, by specialists in quitting smoking. Telephone counselling is much less effective. Even better is to join a group of smokers led by a specialist. It is easier to provide a specialist for several patients than to do so on a one-to-one basis. Equally important, the group increases the support available to each member and as they discuss their difficulties and share useful tips and ideas, the chances of success increase.

The best results, however, are obtained by combining intensive expertly guided supporting a group with some pharmalogical treatment.

Nicotine is the agent inhaled from tobacco in cigarettes. It gets into the bloodstream and stimulates the brain. Although the nicotine in cigarettes is addictive, it is not the nicotine itself but other chemicals in the cigarette that cause most of the damage. It is possible to replace the nicotine supply without the smoke in the form of chewing gum, skin patches, tablets that dissolve under the tongue or by inhalation of nasal sprays. All of these preparations are effective in increasing the number of people who are able to quit.

Another way of dealing with nicotine addiction is to give drugs that interfere with the way that nicotine affects the brain. This is how varenicline (Champix) works. Varenicline limits the effects of nicotine on the body by partly stimulating the brain. This reduces the urge to smoke and relieves withdrawal symptoms. However, at the same time, varenicline blocks the effects of nicotine on the brain, so that the effects of having a cigarette are reduced in those patients who give in to temptation and light a cigarette. Varenicline more than doubles the rate of success in stopping smoking when compared with inactive dummy tablets.

Varenicline is generally thought to be safe. As with all new medicines, however, it must be used with caution. People who are pregnant or breastfeeding, under 18, and those with severe kidney disease should not use it. It may also cause problems in people with mental health disorders and obviously you should check all this out with your doctor before starting it. One difficulty is that it quite often causes minor side-effects, such as nausea or wind, and this may worry patients who are suffering from CD. Often they find that if they take the tablet after a meal, these effects are reduced.

The usual course of treatment with varenicline is 12 weeks but this may be extended to an additional 12 weeks of treatment by your doctor. You will need a prescription to obtain varenicline and you will have had to decide on the date you wish to stop smoking before you start it. You should start taking the tablets one week before that date. This is to build up the dose within your body. The dose is gradually increased until the full amount of 1mg twice daily is reached on the day you intend to stop smoking. Varenicline is then continued at this level for 11 weeks.

If you have not succeeded in stopping smoking after 12 weeks, there is usually no point in continuing with this treatment.

The other drug which may be used to help smokers to give up the habit is bupropion. This drug was initially introduced as an antidepressant and its mode of action in stopping smoking is not clear. It may involve an effect on chemicals in the brain, which are stimulated by nicotine.

Bupropion may cause gastrointestinal side-effects and should not be taken by people who have seizures as it may make this worse. It may impair the performance of tasks such as driving.

Again treatment should start one to two weeks before the target stop date, initially at 150mg daily for six weeks then the full dose of 150mg twice daily for seven to nine weeks. If the patient continues to smoke after seven weeks, the drug should not be continued.

HOW SHOULD I SET ABOUT GIVING UP SMOKING?

A lot depends on what facilities there are available to you locally. You will in any case need to discuss the matter with your doctor who will have to give you the necessary prescriptions. Most surgeries nowadays have specially trained staff who supervise smoking cessation clinics or are able to give personal advice. Some hospitals have clinics available, but by no means all. When one considers how much the damage caused by smoking costs the NHS in Britain, it is very sad that these clinics are not more widely available.

Patients with CD face particular problems in giving up smoking and have difficulties – such as bowel symptoms – that they may be reluctant to discuss in a group of smokers who have altogether different health problems. Given the value of group therapy in quitting, it's a good idea to see if you could get together a group of CD patients who all wish to quit. Perhaps you might find other people willing to try in your local Crohn's and Colitis UK branch? (See page 239.)

This is how a seven-week course to help IBD patients give up smoking works at Addenbrooke's Hospital. The majority of patients will have CD, although as we have mentioned earlier (page 39), it's still a good idea for patients with UC to give up smoking as well. Partners or a close friend who wish to quit are welcomed to the group if all the CD patients are in agreement. The course is held at the hospital in surroundings that are familiar to the patients and the group contains, as well as the specialist in smoking cessation, one of the IBD nurses. The IBD nurse is there to provide information and encouragement and also to deal with any specific gut problems that may arise during the programme, so that those patients don't become discouraged. One session includes an IBD dietitian, as a common problem many smokers face after quitting is weight gain. The dietitian helps to advise on dealing with this problem, particularly in patients who may have food intolerances. Some patients may become constipated as they quit and can be advised on the management of this. In addition, sessions include an introduction to aromatherapy, massage, relaxation and some yoga exercises, but these are helpful rather than essential.

The clinic starts with two weeks of preparation, during which time any medication required, such as nicotine or varenicline, can be started. Problems and anxieties are discussed and the quit date for the group is fixed for a couple of weeks later. One common problem faced in this early phase is patients' anxieties about how they can deal with stress when they can't smoke. It's important to remember that smoking does not relieve stress, but merely provides short-term relief. Patients are advised how to deal with stress in straightforward and much healthier ways.

When 'quit night' arrives in week three, it is often a quiet evening as patients muse on the difficulties they face. It's here where continuing follow-up is seen to be so important.

There are further meetings at weeks four to seven, during which advice and encouragement is provided, and the patients share their experiences and explain how they have got over their own particular difficulties, which may, of course, be very helpful to others.

The success of clinics such as this is such that one can only hope that they may soon become more easily available. If you are really keen to quit smoking yourself, why not try to set up your own group? Discussion with your GP or hospital specialist will point you in the right direction to find the cessation specialist who will be able to guide you along the way to success. The NHS has a free quit-smoking helpline on 0800 022 4332 and provides a quit kit which is available on http://smokefree.nhs.uk

You need to stop smoking and you no doubt know several others who would like to give up as well. Why not get together, form a group and get on with it!

HYGIENE AND IBD

Although IBD is not infectious, it's nevertheless important to avoid anything that may lead to infection and make the condition worse. The most common way to get a bowel infection is from contaminated food. Some general points to remember when cooking and storing food include:

Food preparation: before and after preparing food, wash hands, ensuring nails are clean. Make sure all surfaces for food preparation are cleaned beforehand and do not prepare salads and cooked meats on the same surface as raw meat or use the same utensils without washing between uses. This can cause contamination by bacteria, which would normally be destroyed on cooking. Always wash salads, fruits and veg before eating and keep animals away while preparing food – and wash hands after playing with your pets.

Cooking foods: make sure food is thoroughly cooked, especially meat and poultry. Bacteria can produce spores when in unfavourable conditions such as freezing and can begin to multiply again as conditions became warmer. Do not reheat food. Repeated warming allows ideal conditions for bacterial growth.

Food storage: always cover foods that are left out, to protect them from flies or cross-contamination from other foods. Do not store cooked and uncooked meats together. Cooked meats should always be kept at the top of the fridge and uncooked at the bottom. Ensure that the fridge and freezer are in good working order and that their temperatures are correct (fridge not above 4°C); do not refreeze defrosted or partially defrosted food, and after cooking ensure food is cooled down before putting in the freezer as hot food may begin to defrost other food in the freezer. Do not keep foods longer than is safely recommended.

General points with food: do not eat foods which appear to be 'blown out' or from dented tins and cartons. This could indicate bacterial contamination. Do not eat foods that look, taste or smell different from usual nor those which are out of date.

Unfortunately, stomach upsets do happen occasionally when eating out and it's generally prudent to know the history of the restaurant before you dine there. If someone in the family has an upset stomach, be extra vigilant to prevent it spreading to yourself and others, by fastidious hand washing, using high temperatures for washing dishes and by regular cleaning and disinfection of the lavatory.

EMPLOYMENT

CD and UC are chronic diseases that may flare up from time to time, but with appropriate treatment patients should be asymptomatic and remain well for long periods. There is no reason why a person with IBD cannot enjoy full employment. However, there are certain jobs that might not be ideal for patients who suffer chronic diarrhoea.

Most patients with IBD may feel more confident if they have quick and easy access to a lavatory. Therefore, working as a pilot, train or bus driver, courier or construction worker might cause problems. Most jobs are offered subject to a medical examination and it's wise to be honest from the beginning, gaining sympathy and understanding from an employer, rather than facing dismissal (or even legal action) if the situation becomes difficult later on. A letter from your GP may be required to confirm that you are able to work.

Honesty and openness with colleagues can avoid the necessity for secrecy over following a special diet, taking medicines, running to the loo or having stomach pains. The more your workmates know and understand, the more helpful people will be. Remember, IBD is not infectious and you are not in any way endangering the health of your colleagues.

EMPLOYEE'S RIGHTS

Most people with IBD enjoy a good working life and have the same benefits from a job that are enjoyed by a person without such a problem. However, it is important to be aware of your rights including sick leave and pay, pension rights and job security. If it becomes apparent that you are being discriminated against because of your illness, or for any other reason, you should speak to your human resources department, or equivalent. Problems may have developed with the lack of understanding of the disease on your employer's part and giving them further information or a letter from your doctor may help to ease the problem. If the situation is still difficult, you may be able to consult your union representative or contact the department of employment (www.direct.gov.uk/en/Employment). The Citizens Advice Bureau may be able to help.

EMPLOYER'S RIGHTS

An employer has the right to expect that an employee will perform the job for which he is paid, and when this does not happen, he is legally entitled to terminate the contract. It pays to be honest from the beginning, as your employer cannot be expected to make any allowances for you if he is unaware of your IBD. Equally, he may not have employed you at all if he had considered that you were unsuitable for the post.

Having IBD must not be allowed to stop you from being successful at work or mean that you are less valuable to your employer. If problems arise from time to time, understanding and tolerance from both parties should ensure a smooth, working relationship.

HOLIDAYS AND TRAVEL

We all love going on holiday but we are all well aware that bowel upsets are more likely to occur when we are away. It's therefore important to select your destination sensibly when going on holiday.

Select somewhere suitable: choosing a suitable destination can make the difference between a lovely holiday and disappointment. Holidays in the UK usually pose few problems as the environment is little changed. Holidays abroad are different, however, and destinations renowned to have poor hygiene are best avoided. If you must travel to such places, ensure that your accommodation is of the highest possible standard.

Travel insurance: make sure that you have a comprehensive travel insurance policy before you leave home and that pre-existing medical conditions are not excluded. Do not travel against your doctor's advice as this may make the policy void. A letter from the doctor would be helpful and it may also be useful to have this if you are taking medication or elemental diet with you, to avoid difficulties with customs. Be familiar with the procedure for obtaining medical treatment or making an insurance claim. Remember that in the EU free emergency medical treatment can be obtained by British subjects. For this purpose, the E111 card can be obtained either online or at a post office.

It's best to shop around for the most suitable policy as some companies are more sympathetic than others towards chronic illness.

If you're travelling off the beaten track, it's sensible to have travel insurance that covers medical evacuation to the nearest region with adequate medical facilities if you should be unfortunate enough to become seriously ill.

Mode of transport: this is very important in terms of the availability and accessibility of toilet facilities. Some long-distance coaches have loos on board and it's worth checking before you book. Coaches that take holiday-makers from the airport to their resort usually don't have these and it may be worth checking the transfer time from the airport when deciding on which resort to choose. Most trains, whether in Britain or abroad, have toilets and it's possible sometimes to book a seat near one. Information on toilet facilities at ports and on ferries to the continent is available from the reservations office (or the website). Stena Sealink has advice leaflets containing these details for all its routes.

Air travel can lead to difficulties in gaining quick and easy access to the lavatory. On some airlines it's possible to prebook a seat which is near to the loo or to pay for speedy boarding so you can choose a suitable seat. Most airports have information leaflets (or use their website) giving details of medical centres and the location of toilet facilities.

When travelling by car it is worth remembering that there is a scheme that enables drivers to hold a special key for lavatories that are not available to others. It's therefore unlikely that you will have to wait and these toilets are unlikely to be dirty or vandalised. To purchase or hire one of these keys contact the Royal Association for Disability and Rehabilitation (RADAR) tel: 0207 250 3222 (www.radar.org.uk).

MEDICATION

Ensure that you have an adequate supply of any medications you are taking as you may have difficulties in replenishing these if you run short on holiday. Medications should be kept in your hand luggage for easy availability. Your doctor will be able to give you advice on the use of short-term anti-diarrhoeal treatments to avoid accidents while travelling, although, of course, the regular use of such medication is not generally recommended as they can lead to complications of IBD. However, a tablet of codeine or Imodium may give you more confidence as you set out. Your doctor may also give you advice on increasing your medication should you suffer a flare-up while away.

FOOD AND DRINK

A change in environment may affect your tolerance to foods, and so you should be vigilant while abroad. In general you should not eat anything you would not eat at home because exotic and highly spiced foods may upset your gut. If you are going to a hot country it's sensible to keep to the following recommendations:

> Increase your fluid and salt intake so as to avoid dehydration

> Check if the local tap water is safe to drink; in general it's better to use bottled water for drinking and teeth cleaning – make sure the bottle's seal is not broken

> Avoid ice cubes as they are usually made from tap water

> Choose freshly cooked food whenever possible and avoid cold foods and ice cream

> If you are self-catering, salads and fruit should be washed in bottled water before eating

The inside of fruit is usually sterile, but you should peel all fresh fruit yourself. The beautiful fruit displays at some hotels make tempting targets for flies!

If your CD is being treated by diet, take a small supply of elemental diet with you. As noted above, your doctor may need to give you a short note about this in order to avoid difficulties at customs.

PREVENTATIVE MEDICINE AND TRAVEL ABROAD

Travel outside EU often leads to the need for vaccinations or medications against conditions such as malaria. Your GP will be able to advise you about this.

Special precautions need to be considered if you are taking a medication that reduces your immune responses, e.g. corticosteroids, 5-ASA or azathioprine. A patient would be considered to be immunosuppressed if he has taken steroids at a dose of over 40mg a day for more than a week, or at a lower dosage or with other immuno-suppressants for a longer period of time.

Patients who are immunosuppressed should not receive live vaccines until at least three months after that treatment has ceased, or been reduced to levels that are not considered to be immunosuppressive. Inactivated vaccines are not dangerous to patients who are immunosuppressed, but the body's response may be reduced and sometimes insufficient to provide complete protection.

Some patients with IBD find that they are upset by anti-malarial tablets. It's best to try these before you leave and it may be possible for your GP to give you a different preparation. However, the risks of contracting malaria in some countries is so high that it is essential that anti-malarial medication is continued throughout your visit and usually for four weeks after your return.

Immunocompromised patients should carry a letter detailing their condition and treatment, and if possible a contact number for the physician who is in charge of their care.

SPORT, EXERCISE AND IBD

Most patients with IBD can enjoy a wide range of sporting activities. Exercise is a good way to improve energy levels and relieve any tendencies to depression because it leads to the release of endorphins, natural feel-good hormones.

Some conditions may limit strenuous activity. If you have had a relapse and are suffering active disease you won't feel in a sporting mood and in general it's better to rest. Fears of incontinence and anxiety that loos are not easily available may also discourage you. However, the aim is to have treatment that is so effective that you can resume exercise as soon as possible.

Osteoporosis may mean that vigorous exercise is best avoided. Exercise may help to strengthen the bones and preserve their structure, but bones break more easily when they are osteoporotic. It's therefore customary to advise against certain sports such as heavy gym work, football, rugby or hockey. Patients with osteoporosis are recommended to try swimming (where the body is supported by the water), water aerobics, stretch-and-tone exercises such as yoga and pilates, golf, cycling and walking.

Vigorous sports should be avoided after recent surgery. When the wounds have healed, it is generally possible to restart your fitness activities. Ask your doctor's advice. The presence of a stoma need not prevent most forms of exercise. This is discussed in chapter 8.

INSURANCE AND IBD

Most applications for insurance, whether it is life insurance, a mortgage application or pension plan, are subject to a medical questionnaire. People with chronic illnesses, including IBD, may find that they have to pay a higher premium in order to obtain satisfactory cover.

This may seem unfair as studies have shown that the long-term prognosis for patients with IBD has improved so much over recent decades that expectation of life is virtually normal. There is an increase of colorectal carcinoma, but in other respects IBD has generally been felt to have little effect on mortality. Premiums continue to be loaded because insurance companies complain that the death rate in patients with IBD is slightly higher than would be expected for people of that age and social status.

Shop around to find the company which will give you the best deal. It may be useful to seek help from an independent professional insurance broker who has access to a range of companies and may know of those that are sympathetic to IBD and have sufficient experience to rate your risk fairly.

When filling in an application for insurance it's important to be honest about your medical status as failure to disclose information might cause the policy to be invalid. It also helps to be quite specific about your disease. Do not say UC if you only have proctitis. Proctitis carries no increased risk of cancer and this should be reflected in the premium that you pay. Policies may also be rated for surgical interventions, the types of treatments employed and the number of relapses.

Some companies may request a medical examination before they will consider providing cover. Such an examination is always at their expense and they will usually appoint an independent doctor to perform it.

If your IBD is well controlled and you can get your GP or hospital to support you, there is no reason why you should be heavily penalised. You should be able to obtain a policy with affordable premiums providing adequate cover for you and your family.

The official insurance advisor to Crohn's and Colitis UK is:

CBG Financial Services
Southmoor House
Southmoor Road
Manchester
M23 9XD

Telephone: 01616 200 200
www.cbg-group.co.uk

This company can offer advice on life insurance, pensions, savings and investments, etc. Unlimited medical expenses and emergency services are offered as part of travel insurance to Crohn's and Colitis UK members.

GENETICS AND IBD

The role of genetics in the pathogenesis of IBD has been discussed in chapter 2. CD tends to run in families and people who have a first-degree relative with IBD have a 10% risk of contracting the disease. This does not mean, however, that people with IBD should not have children. The risk of their children developing CD is 10%; this implies that there is a 90% chance they will not. The treatment of IBD is steadily improving and if you would like to have a family, there is no reason why you should not go ahead.

SEXUALITY

Active IBD is almost inevitably associated with reduction in libido, but overall the fertility of patients with IBD is relatively normal.

Sex itself, however, may present some problems. In one study it was found that six times as many women with CD preferred to avoid sex, than did matched controls. More encouragingly, in those women who did have sex, there was no reduction in frequency and enjoyment. There are three main problems. The first is that some women have pain during intercourse. This is often the result of active inflammation and if there is no gynaecological abnormality, painful intercourse in women may be an indication for intestinal surgery if medical measures are not effective.

The fear of the embarrassment of faecal incontinence is a major factor affecting both men and women. This is something that does not happen as much as may be feared, but nevertheless is sufficient to put some people completely off the idea of forming any potentially sexual relationship. As with travel, an anti-diarrhoeal tablet taken before intercourse may provide sufficient reassurance. Finally, the presence of a stoma may be an off-putting factor. For this reason, most physicians try and avoid the creation of the stoma in patients who are young and single, but experience shows that established partners usually deal with the problem successfully. Advice from your stoma care nurse may be very useful here.

When a vaginal discharge is a consequence of a recto-vaginal fistula, fortunately something that is quite rare, the use of a condom may be very helpful. If the couple are looking to start a family, a vaginal douche before intercourse may be the answer. As always, talk to your GP if you have any worries about having sex while your IBD is active.

PREGNANCY AND IBD

IBD does not affect the outcome of pregnancy and more than 80% of affected women are able to carry healthy babies to full term. Occasionally, previous surgery, and in particular ileo-anal pouches, may lead obstetricians to recommend delivery by C-section rather than vaginal delivery.

The risk of miscarriage and congenital abnormalities is no greater in patients with IBD than that of patients without. Patients with severe disease requiring surgery have an increased risk of obstetric complications, but with the use of intravenous feeding, the outcome has been increasingly successful.

THE EFFECT OF PREGNANCY ON PATIENTS WITH IBD

Most patients find that their IBD goes into remission during pregnancy and they feel very well. This is particularly true in patients with CD, and I attribute this to being an effect of the high levels of female sex hormones, namely oestrogen and progesterone, during pregnancy. This appears to have an immunosuppressive effect and flare-ups are less common. Patients on a diet for CD usually find that they can eat more widely during pregnancy. They must, however, take care when the baby is born and hormone levels fall. There is then a risk that the disease will flare up if they continue to eat foods that had previously upset them but were safe during pregnancy. After delivery, it is important to return to the established diet.

Overall the risk of the disease relapsing during pregnancy is about a third, which is no higher than the risk of relapse in patients who are not pregnant. Relapses tend to be more common in the first three months and can be severe following delivery, possibly due to a sudden fall in hormone levels.

The course of the disease during pregnancy usually relates to disease activity at the time of conception. Therefore, it's best to try to avoid becoming pregnant when the disease is active.

Ileostomy patients may have trouble with the function of the stoma in the second trimester due to displacement by the growing baby: 10% are reported to have some degree of obstruction, which means that 90% are perfectly okay. Obstruction means that abdominal pain develops and the stoma ceases to function. You should contact your doctor immediately.

THE EFFECTS OF DRUGS ON PREGNANCY AND THE FOETUS

Most drugs used in the treatment of IBD are relatively safe for use during pregnancy and the reported incidence of abnormalities to the baby are no higher than would be expected in the general population. Supplements of folic acid are recommended before and during pregnancy, especially when patients are taking sulphasalazine, which causes levels to fall in the body. Patients taking methotrexate should not become pregnant. Certain antibiotics such as metronidazole should not be used in the first trimester of pregnancy and thereafter only for severe peri-anal disease. Most antibiotics also tend to pass into breast milk, but it is usually not necessary to stop breast-feeding as the levels in breast milk are less than the usual doses prescribed for infants.

INVESTIGATIONS DURING PREGNANCY

X-rays must be avoided during pregnancy. Fortunately, as the majority of patients experience a remission of disease during pregnancy, this is rarely an issue. Ultrasound scans are quite harmless, as is MRI. White-cell scans involve little exposure to radiation and may be useful to monitor disease progress in pregnancy.

ORAL CONTRACEPTION

There has been considerable debate about the role of oral contraceptives in IBD. Initial suggestions that they might make it worse were contested because the role of smoking was not fully taken into account. However, a small number of women found that their IBD improved when they came off the Pill. A recent study from London suggested that the risk of developing IBD, corrected for smoking, was increased one and a half times in women on the Pill even if they were taking low-dose preparations. This is too small an effect really to be troublesome and I would never stop my patients taking it.

However, IBD may cause difficulties in taking the Pill. The Pill is 99% effective if taken correctly; however, in IBD its absorption may be reduced. This could be because the surface of the intestine has been damaged by inflammation and ulceration. Diarrhoea may lead to a faster speed of transit through the bowel, which may reduce absorption, and previous surgery may lessen the absorptive surface available. Medications may interfere with absorption of the Pill – for example, antibiotics may lead to diarrhoea. For these reasons it may be necessary to take a higher-dose Pill to ensure its effectiveness.

It is strongly advised that additional methods of contraception such as condoms or caps are also used at times when absorption of the Pill may be impaired, such as when disease activity is increased or when taking drugs that may cause diarrhoea.

In some cases the Pill may prove not to be sufficiently reliable and it may necessary to discuss alternative methods of contraception with your doctor or family planning clinic.

OSTEOPOROSIS

Osteoporosis is a condition resulting in loss of protein and calcium from bone, causing the bones to become weak and thin and thus increasing the risk of fracture. The main cause of osteoporosis is the long-term use of corticosteroids (see page 166). Anyone who has taken more than 5g of prednisolone over a long course of time is likely to suffer from loss of bone density. There is some evidence that disease activity may also make osteoporosis worse, but this may be merely a reflection of the corticosteroid use to control it. It may also be important that absorption of vitamin D and calcium may be reduced in the presence of diarrhoea or a damaged small intestine.

Osteoporosis may be suspected on X-rays of the bones, but the main investigation to prove its presence is the determination of bone density (page 77). In complex cases and particularly if there is thought to be significant vitamin D malabsorption as well, a bone biopsy from the iliac crest – the upper edge of the pelvic bone, may also be necessary.

Nowadays, osteoporosis is treatable but the emphasis should still be on prevention rather than cure. All patients who are on steroids should take generous calcium and vitamin D supplements such as Calcichew tablets twice daily or if the dose of steroids is above 10mg, Calcichew D3 twice daily. All patients on a diet for CD, who are unable to take dairy products, should also take calcium supplements.

Exercise is very good for building up strong bones and prevents mineral loss at any age. With increasing age contact sports are best avoided. Swimming, however, is an excellent all-round exercise that puts very little stress on the muscles and bones of the body. Gym sessions, cycling and walking are also excellent exercises.

Some doctors recommend HRT (hormone replacement therapy) in post-menopausal women as a way of reducing the risks of osteoporosis. This is somewhat controversial as HRT may slightly increase the risk of uterine and breast cancer. Furthermore, there is an increased risk of venous thrombosis. Many women feel so much better on HRT that they are quite prepared to run these small risks. Clearly it's sensible to discuss this with your doctor who will be able to take your own individual factors into consideration.

Biphosphonates are drugs which are effective in preventing post-menopausal osteoporosis and which also may reverse existing bone damage. These drugs are absorbed into the bone and attach themselves to bone crystals slowing both their rate of growth, but more importantly their rate of dissolution and therefore reducing the rate of bone turnover. Biphosphonates may upset the bowel and this sometimes means that they have to be given intravenously. They may also cause trouble in the jaws, and patients who take these should take great care to keep their teeth clean. Ideally any important dental work should be completed before biphosphonates are started.

In established cases of osteoporosis other treatments including calcitonin, strontium ranelate and teriparatide may necessary. These should be discussed with your doctor.

CONSTIPATION

Constipation is when stools take too long to pass through the bowel. This means that the bowels are open infrequently, perhaps less than three times per week. It also can mean that the stools are small, hard and dry. It may be necessary to strain hard to pass them and there may be discomfort, abdominal pain and bloating. Most people with IBD suffer diarrhoea rather than constipation, but occasionally constipation is a real problem. This is particularly true of patients with left-sided colitis and proctitis. They may develop proximal constipation – that is to say, faeces may collect on the right side of the bowel. For reasons that we don't understand, this seems to make the UC worse. It's often necessary to clear out the bowel completely before the inflammation will heal. Constipation often appears to be a factor leading to relapse of IBD and therefore when you are in remission it's best to try and avoid it if at all possible.

One of the main functions of the large intestine is to reabsorb water from food residues that pass along it following digestion. If too much water is taken out the motion becomes hard, small and difficult to pass. This may arise from a number of reasons. A poor diet, low in fibre-rich foods, provides insufficient residue and, if fluid intake is insufficient, drying of stools in the large intestine becomes a bigger problem. A sedentary lifestyle and lack of exercise may also lead to constipation. Certain medications, such as painkillers, antacids and antidepressants, may cause constipation, which may be a sign of more important complications of IBD such as stricture or even cancer. A detailed consideration of constipation and its management is given in the companion volume *Irritable Bowel Solutions* (Vermilion, 2007).

When patients are in remission, treatment of constipation is usually fairly straightforward. It's important that the diet contains adequate amounts of fruit and vegetables with wholegrain cereal products such as brown rice or wholemeal bread to produce larger and softer stools that can be passed without difficulty. If food intolerance is a problem it is usually a good idea to take a non-fermentable bulk laxative such as cracked linseed or Normacol to increase stool volume. Fibre intake should be increased gradually to ensure that it does not produce too much wind and to ensure that fluid intake remains adequate. Increasing fibre without increasing fluid may actually make constipation worse. Remember that coffee, tea and alcoholic beverages may have the effect of making you pass more urine, and therefore becoming somewhat dehydrated. It's better to drink water and soft drinks and to ensure that the daily intake is at least two litres.

Exercise as much as you can, particularly if your work is largely sedentary. If you spend much of the day sitting or crouched over your desk, ensure that you are more active when you get home. Walk instead of using the car wherever possible and get into the habit of using the stairs instead of the lift. And have brief but regular breaks in which you can walk round your office or place of work.

Try to develop a good bowel habit. When the stomach is filled there is a reflex that causes the bowel to contract. This is called the gastro-colic reflex and is a natural urge to empty the bowel, which is usually strongest after breakfast. Take advantage of this to make sure that your habit becomes regular.

Sometimes laxatives are essential. There are four main groups of these. Bulking agents are usually the simplest and the best and it's better if they are not fermented, as this means they are less likely to give you wind. They absorb water causing swelling and an increase in the stool matter and it is moved more easily along the bowel. They need to be used with care in the presence of intestinal strictures.

Sometimes lubricants help. Examples are liquid paraffin and glycerine. These work by allowing the stool to slide more easily along the bowel.

Osmotic agents include Epsom salts, lactulose and mannitol. These increase the osmotic pressure of the gut contents and draw water into the intestine. This in turn increases stool volume and softness. Some, particularly lactulose, which is poorly absorbed and passes down to the gut bacteria, may increase fermentation with undesirable side-effects.

Finally, there are bowel stimulants such as senna and syrup of figs. These stimulate the bowel muscles to help propel stools more vigorously along. Unfortunately, if used regularly in the long term, their effects may start to wear off and you may have to increase the dose in order for them to be as effective.

Most of my patients find that their bowels are well controlled if they take a daily bulk laxative such as cracked linseed or Normacol washed down with plenty of water. Some of them in addition require a dose of stimulant laxative such as senna once or twice a week.

It may seem that life with IBD becomes extremely complex and difficult. This is not the case. Many of the possible problems mentioned will not affect you personally and as you gain more experience of dealing with your IBD these will become everyday matters that cause you little concern. It is quite common, when I ask patients with CD how their diet is progressing, for them to reply: 'What diet?' When questioned further they will say, 'Oh, of course, I never eat oats or cheese.' This has become such second nature to them that they have quite forgotten that they have any dietary restrictions! Life for IBD sufferers can still be great fun.

CHAPTER 10

Probiotics and prebiotics

PROBIOTICS

Probiotics are 'living' bacteria that when taken in sufficient numbers produce health benefits beyond their simple nutritional or pharmacological value, such as relieving diarrhoea or excess flatulence.

The theory that probiotic bacteria might improve health has been around for a long time. The Russian Nobel Prize-winning scientist Eli Metchnikoff first suggested that some people in Central Europe were enjoying very long lives due to the habit of drinking fermented milk that had been turned sour by bacteria such as *lactobacilli* and *bifidobacter*. Metchnikoff was not able to confirm this theory, but in recent years there has been an explosion of interest in the possible health benefits of taking healthy non-pathogenic bacteria.

It all sounds very simple but in reality the use of probiotic bacteria is quite difficult. If you look round health food shops and some supermarkets, you will find the shelves contain many strains of bacteria (sometimes in the form of yoghurt) that are promoted as providing benefits to health. When we first started looking into this matter many years ago, we found that in many of these products the bacteria were in fact dead. The process of growing, purifying and then freeze-drying had been too much and no bacterial activity remained. Clearly, this could be of very little benefit.

A successful probiotic organism is rather special. It must possess the following characteristics:

✓ Must not cause disease

✓ Must not contain any toxins

✓ Must be resistant to the effects of acid (so it can pass through the stomach without being destroyed)

✓ Must be resistant to the effects of alkalis, bile salts and digestive enzymes in the small bowel

✓ Must be able to compete with resident bacteria living in lower bowel

✓ Must be able to attach itself to the bowel lining so it is not swept straight out

✓ Must produce chemicals (known as bacteriocins) that repel other bacteria allowing it to survive

Once in the gut, probiotic bacteria might have beneficial effects in a number of ways. As well as perhaps reducing fermentation in the intestine, they might suppress inflammation, help break down bile acids or reduce the secretion of mucus and fluids into the gut. They might affect other bacteria by inhibiting enzymes or competing for bacterial nutrients. They might repel other bacteria by the production of bacteriocins and stop other bacteria attaching themselves to the lining of the gut or invading body tissues. They might tighten the junction between cells so as to reduce the chances of bacteria passing through.

The known interaction between the gut bacteria and the immune system might suggest that IBD was an ideal condition in which to try out probiotic bacteria. Although no convincing specific pathogen has yet been isolated in IBD, the gut flora is clearly abnormal. In UC, the numbers of *bifidobacter* are much reduced and there is an overgrowth of facultative anaerobes, oxygen-loving bacteria that somehow contrive to survive in the large bowel where oxygen is in short supply. The intestinal bacteria in CD have not yet been fully documented, but again there is an increase in unusual species of facultative anaerobes.

COLONISATION RESISTANCE

One of the difficulties with probiotic bacteria is colonisation resistance. This is one of the body's defence mechanisms. The gut of a baby is sterile when the infant is born. Bacteria start to colonise the gut during the very process of birth, the baby meeting some of its mother's bacteria even as it passes down the birth canal (the gut microflora in a baby born by Caesarean section is at first less complex than those born in the natural way).

Breast-feeding encourages the development of a healthy gut flora. Indeed recent research has suggested that helpful bacteria like *lactobacilli* are absorbed from the mother's bowel and secreted in the breast milk itself so that the baby gets a good supply of them. How is it that these bacteria are not destroyed by the immune system?

During the first three months of life the infant's immune system does not react at all. This is known as immune tolerance. A tiny number of babies may need a liver transplant at this stage, but if so, immunosuppressive drugs are not needed to prevent the new liver being rejected – the transplanted organ is accepted by the immune system as 'self', as if it were a normal part of the infant's body. It is likely that the purpose of immune tolerance is to enable the baby to establish a population of bacteria in the large intestine. Those bacteria that the baby meets during that period are accepted as 'self' and survive.

When the baby is a few weeks old, however, the window of immune tolerance closes and thereafter any bacteria that are not already recognised by the immune system as 'self' are vigorously rejected and cannot establish themselves permanently in the gut flora. This phenomenon is called 'colonisation resistance', and it means that the gut flora remains very stable during healthy adult life.

It follows that although any bacteria that the infant encounters in the early weeks of life will be regarded as normal members of the bacterial flora for the rest of that person's life, it is not possible to correct and maintain simply by taking preparations of probiotics. Unless the organism has been encountered in infancy in health, it will not colonise the gut.

Interesting indirect support for this theory was recently published. It had been shown that if mothers in late pregnancy and infants at birth were given the probiotic agent *Lactobacillus casei* GG, the incidence of allergic diseases in the infants during early childhood was reduced. In one study in which this organism was given to mothers and children for this purpose, the bacterium was found to disappear from the stools of the mothers as soon as they stopped taking it. In the infants, however, it was still present two years later, implying that it had become established as part of their normal flora, although not in those of their mothers.

PROBIOTICS IN IBD

The choice of a suitable organism to act as a probiotic is not easy and it must be admitted that, to date, there is little, if any, evidence that it is possible to change the course of CD by using probiotics. In UC, however, the picture is not quite so gloomy.

During the First World War, German physician Professor Alfred Nissle noted that some of the soldiers in the German army appeared to be more resistant to the infectious diarrhoea that was so common in the trenches than were their comrades. This intrigued him and he isolated a number of organisms from the stools of these 'resistant' soldiers. These were then tested to see how they affected the growth of the bacterium which causes typhus. The organism which had the most dramatic effect was *Escherichia coli* (Nissle, 1979). Professor Nissle tried taking this organism himself and when he found that it produced no ill-effects, he called it Mutaflor and, supplied in a capsule that is resistant to stomach acid, it has been on sale in Europe ever since to protect against gastroenteritis.

Mutaflor has since been used in three separate studies of UC and in each it has been found that it's as effective as mesalazine (pages 138, 148–149) in preventing relapse.

In separate studies similar results were obtained using another organism *Lactobacillus rhamnosus* GG and also by giving milk fermented by the addition of bifidobacteria. Some of my patients claim great benefit from a pro-biotic mixture called CP-1 available from gut doctor (www.gutdoctor.com). They are expensive and I know of no formal trial confirming their value.

However, the therapeutic benefit of a single species or strain of bacteria will clearly be limited and it has now been suggested that a mixture of several organisms may prove more effective. VSL-#3 is such a preparation. It contains 450 billion bacteria in every dose and these are a mixture of eight different species. There are three different bifidobacteria (*B.longum*, *B.infantis*, *B.brevis*), four different lactobacilli (*L.acidophilus*, *L.casei*, *L.bulgaricus*, *L.plantarum*) and also *Streptococcus salivarius* subspecies *thermophilus*. There have now been a number of successful trials of this mixture in UC. Perhaps the best results are seen in pouchitis, where administration of VSL-#3 after a course of antibiotics is an effective way of settling the inflammation, which is also less likely to recur if VSL-#3 is continued.

VSL-#3 has also been shown not only to reduce the rate of relapse in patients with UC, but also to be effective in producing remission in mild to moderately active cases. As a result of these studies, VSL-#3 is now available on NHS prescription in the UK.

POSSIBLE FUTURE DEVELOPMENTS

The results in UC are such that we have reason to be optimistic about the future value of probiotics in IBD. True, there are no trials as yet that provide convincing evidence of their value in CD, but this is almost certainly because we have not yet sorted out the ideal way to use them.

We are more likely to be successful when we have found ways of breaking colonisation resistance. This must be possible, for we get overgrowth of bacteria in a number of conditions such as, for example, pseudomembraneous colitis, where there is overgrowth of *Clostridium difficile*, which may be quite difficult to treat. Possible ways of breaking colonisation resistance include diet and antibiotics. Either of these, combined with a good probiotic preparation, would be worth trialling in IBD.

From the example of VSL-#3, it would seem that it is likely that probiotic mixtures made up of many different types of bacteria will prove more effective than a single species. This has been taken to its logical conclusion by some doctors who have given enemas of faeces from healthy individuals to some patients with UC. There are a number of reports in which such an approach has provided long-lasting remission. This approach has yet to catch on. Partly this is because of the understandable reluctance of health professionals to work with such unpleasant material as faeces! And it's also because one is never quite sure what one may be giving. While the faeces might merely be full of hundreds of healthy bacteria, it is quite possible that it might contain an unknown pathogen.

When one considers the precautions we have to take nowadays to avoid transmission of disease such as hepatitis and CJD, to instil someone else's faeces into another person's body sounds foolhardy. Ideally, like Professor Nissle, one would isolate healthy bacteria from faeces and grow them in the laboratory. Pure growths might then be mixed together before being given to the patient. The difficulty here is that we can only grow 60% of the bacteria that are present in our bowels and the ones that we cannot isolate may be the ones that provide the benefit. Furthermore, bacteria are living organisms that are constantly adapting to their environment. When they are grown in the lab, away from the turbulent conditions of the human colon, they may change in subtle ways and repeated episodes of growth in the lab may reduce their effectiveness.

The suppliers of VSL-#3 have got round this problem by setting up a store of thousands of samples of the original successful culture which are kept in the deep freeze until they are required. Thus their nature will not change and they can be assured that the original quality will be retained. Despite these difficulties, it's clear that further research into probiotics for IBD will continue apace.

PREBIOTICS

Probiotics provide healthy bacteria in the hope of improving the gut flora. Another approach is to feed the bacteria with substances that may encourage the growth of the bacteria whose numbers need to be increased.

Such substances need to pass along the small intestine without being digested so that they are available for fermentation by the bacteria when they reach the large bowel. These substances are known as prebiotics and they have the great theoretical attraction of being likely to increase the growth of bacteria which are already part of the gut flora and which therefore will not have to contend with the immunological difficulties of colonisation resistance.

The best-known prebiotics are a selection of various complex sugars. Good examples are inulin and fructose-oligosaccharides, which are found in chicory, Jerusalem artichokes, bananas, leeks, asparagus, onions and garlic. The well-known laxative lactulose is also a prebiotic as it passes undigested down to the large bowel. Another source is germinated barley foodstuffs, which is similar to malt.

Prebiotics have been shown to increase the growth of bifidobacteria whose numbers, as we have seen, are often reduced in IBD as well as in other gut disorders. When I first heard of prebiotics I was very excited, as my studies with various probiotics, to try and surmount food intolerances in IBS and CD, had all floundered on colonisation resistance. You could isolate the bacteria from the stools while treatment was continuing, but a fortnight after it was stopped, they disappeared completely.

We have performed a formal trial of 6g of fructose-oligosaccharide a day in patients with IBS. The results were very disappointing. Many patients complained of an unpleasant increase in wind and discomfort. I have no doubt that prebiotics may increase the number and the activity of bifidobacteria in the gut, but they nearly always increase the activity of other bacteria as well. This is the reason that I don't recommend lactulose as a laxative in patients with CD.

Successful treatments of CD such as diet and antibiotics appear to be effective because they reduce the amount of fermentation which is occurring. It therefore seems illogical to give substances to these patients that increase fermentation. Probiotics perhaps, but prebiotics seem unlikely to be of great value. A recent trial in London of fructose-oligosaccharide in CD showed no benefit, which is exactly what I would have predicted!

TRYING PRE- OR PROBIOTICS

If you would like to try a pre- or probiotic and have identified one that you think might be of good quality and likely to be suitable, it's best to discuss this plan with your doctor. People who are very ill and with a weakened immune system, perhaps from high doses of corticosteroids or immunosuppressants, may be at a higher risk of infection from a probiotic. Such infections are very uncommon with only a handful of cases reported out of the many thousands of people who have tried them, but it's best to be aware of the risks.

The side-effects of probiotics are few and far between. Nevertheless, it's a good idea to get your doctor interested in the whole concept before you start. He can point out any possible snags before you trip over them yourself and he will no doubt be very interested to learn of your progress as he is unlikely to have much experience himself in this field. Perhaps the most sensible way forward is to try to persuade him to give you a prescription for VSL-#3 for a month and see what benefit you gain. If you improve, you can carry on with treatment but if, after a month, there is no benefit it's silly to go on longer.

CHAPTER 11

Conclusions

I once looked after a French lady while she was living in England. She had Crohn's disease and did very well on her diet, and she remains well now, many years later. Eventually she decided to move back to France with her family, where she set up an agency for language tuition and translation. She was amazed to discover that people in France seemed to be very surprised that someone who had CD could ever be fit enough to work at all – it was far too unpleasant a condition. She's now trying hard to persuade her compatriots that diet in CD is often the answer!

A negative approach to IBD is what we must try to dispel. IBD *is* treatable. For this reason I never describe my IBD patients as 'disabled'. Yes, of course, it is easy to give up and become a chronic invalid, sitting back and accepting each further relapse, each complication, each operation as stoically as possible. But another of my patients undertook a two-week trek in the Himalayas (taking some enteral feed in her knapsack, just in case!) in order to raise money for her favourite charity.

I want my patients to live life to the full – to get out there and enjoy themselves, take on interesting and rewarding careers, play sport and travel and never accept limitations imposed by IBD.

IBD is a complex condition, and the treatment varies from one case to another. But if you understand what your problem is, and what is available to correct it, you should not rest (and not let your doctor rest!) until you have got it completely under control. It is necessary to pay attention to detail, to try new approaches until you find the one that works, but never be tempted to give up!

I hope very much that this book will help you on your way. IBD can be completely controlled. Good luck!

Useful contacts

Arthritis Care
The UK's largest charity working with and for all people who have arthritis
18 Stephenson Way, London NW1 2HD
020 7380 6500
info@arthritiscare.org.uk
www.arthritiscare.org.uk

British Liver Trust
The national charity working to reduce the impact of liver disease in the UK through support, information, and research
2 Southampton Road, Ringwood BH24 1HY
0800 652 7330
info@britishlivertrust.org.uk
www.britishlivertrust.org.uk

Crohn's and Colitis UK
Formerly The National Association for Colitis and Crohn's Disease, this charity aims to improve life for everyone affected by IBD
4 Beaumont House, Sutton Road, St Albans, Hertfordshire AL1 5HH
0845 130 2233 or +44 (0) 1727 844 296
info@CrohnsAndColitis.org.uk
www.nacc.org.uk

Crohn's in Childhood Research Association
A charity dedicated to creating a wider understanding of CD and UC, particularly as it affects children and young adults
Parkgate House, 356 West Barnes Lane, Motspur Park, Surrey KT3 6NB
020 8949 6209
support@cicra.org
www.cicra.org

crohns.org.uk (website only)
A resource for the management and treatment of Crohn's Disease and other IBDs, designed to help both patients and healthcare professionals

IA (The ileostomy and internal pouch support group)
A UK charity and mutual support group helping those who have had their colon removed
Peverill House, 1–5 Mill Road, Ballyclare, Co. Antrim BT39 9DR
0800 0184 724 (free) or 028 9334 4043
info@iasupport.org
iasupport.org

National Ankylosing Spondylitis Society (NASS)
A UK charity working for people with AS and their families
Unit 0.2, One Victoria Villas, Richmond, Surrey TW9 2GW
020 8948 9117
admin@nass.co.uk
www.nass.co.uk

National Osteoporosis Society
A UK charity dedicated to improving the diagnosis, prevention and treatment of osteoporosis and offering services to those who are concerned about osteoporosis
Camerton, Bath BA2 0PJ
01761 471 771 or 0845 130 3076
Helpline: 0845 450 0230
info@nos.org.uk
www.nos.org.uk

RADAR
The UK's largest disability campaigning organisation
12 City Forum, 250 City Road, London EC1V 8AF
020 7250 3222
radar@radar.org.uk
www.radar.org.uk

Glossary

abscess A localised collection of pus in a cavity formed by the decay of diseased tissues.

acute Sudden onset of symptoms (as in relapse).

aetiology Cause.

anaemia A reduction in the number of red cells, haemoglobin (iron) or volume of packed red cells in the body.

anal fissure A tear or cut near the anus.

anastomosis The joining together of two ends of a healthy bowel after a diseased bowel has been cut out (resected) by the surgeon.

ankylosing spondylitis Chronic inflammatory disease of the spine and nearby joints, which can cause pain and stiffness in the spine, neck, hips, jaw and ribcage.

anus The opening to the back passage.

arthralgia Pains in the joints without swelling.

arthritis Inflammation of a joint(s) with pain, swelling and stiffness.

ascending colon The portion of bowel extending from the caecum to the hepatic flexure.

biopsy Removal of small pieces of tissue from parts of the body (e.g. colon – colonic biopsy) for examination under the microscope for diagnosis.

bowels Another name for the intestines.

caecum The first part of the large intestine forming a dilated pouch into which opens the ileum, the colon and the appendix.

chronic Symptoms occurring over a long period of time.

cobblestoning Characteristic appearance of the bowel

mucosa (lining) seen in Crohn's disease (like 'cobble-stones') formed from deep ulceration and swelling of the surrounding tissue.

colectomy Surgical removal of the colon.

colitis Inflammation of the lining of the colon.

colon The large intestine extending from the caecum to the rectum. It has an ascending, transverse and descending portion.

colonoscopy Inspection of the colon by an illuminated telescope called a colonoscope.

colostomy Surgical creation of an opening between the colon and the surface of the body. Part of the colon is brought out on to the abdomen creating a stoma. A bag is placed over this to collect waste material.

constipation Infrequent bowel motions or difficulty in their passage.

Crohn's disease (CD) A chronic inflammatory disease that can affect the whole of the alimentary tract from the mouth to the anus.

DALM a dysplasia-associated lesion or mass.

defecation The act of passing faeces.

descending colon The portion of bowel between the splenic flexure and the sigmoid colon.

diarrhoea An increase in frequency, urgency, liquidity and weight of bowel motions.

dietary fibre A general term for non-digestible carbohy-drate in food, mostly derived from plant cell walls.

distal Further down the bowel towards the anus.

diverticulum (plural: diverticula) Small pouch-like projec-tions through the muscular wall of the intestine, which may become infected, causing diverticulitis.

duodenum The first part of the small intestine.

dysplasia Alteration in size, shape and organisation of mature cells that indicate the possible development of cancer.

electrolytes Salts in the blood, e.g. sodium, potassium, calcium.

elemental diet Nutritional liquid providing simple components that require no further digestion and are readily absorbed.

embolism Blockage of an artery by a blood clot, which has travelled from further along the blood vessel.

endoscope An instrument for viewing the interior of a body cavity or organ (endoscopy).

endoscopy A collective name for all visual inspections of body cavities with an illuminated telescope. Examples are:
- Gastroscopy
- Colonoscopy
- Sigmoidoscopy

enema A liquid (e.g. barium or steroid) introduced into the rectum for treatment or diagnostic purposes to stimulate the production of a bowel motion.

enteral feeding Where the patient receives nutrition as a liquid feed, often of special composition, which may be taken by mouth, or sometimes through the nose via a naso-gastric tube, or directly into the stomach through the abdominal wall via a percutaneous endoscopic gastrostomy (PEG).

episcleritis Inflammation of the white of the eye and the skin of the eyelashes.

erythema nodosum Red, tender swellings occasionally seen on the shins and lower legs during a flare-up of inflammatory bowel disease. They usually subside when the disease is in remission.

erythrocytes Red cells in the blood which carry oxygen in haemoglobin.

exacerbation An aggravation of symptoms.

faeces The waste matter eliminated from the anus (other names: stools, motions, poo).

fibre optic Flexible fibres which carry light, e.g. in a colonoscope.

fissure A cleft or groove (crack) in the skin surface (e.g. in the anus – anal fissure).

fistula An abnormal connection, usually between two organs, or leading from an internal organ to the body surface (e.g. between the anus and skin surface – anal fistula).

flatus Gas from the rectum.

fulminant colitis Colitis occurring suddenly with great intensity and severity.

gastroenteritis Inflammation of the stomach and intestine, usually caused by infectious bacteria or viruses, leading to vomiting, fever, abdominal pain and diarrhoea.

granulomas Microscopic nodules of cells that can be found in the bowel wall. If present, they strongly suggest Crohn's disease.

gut Another name for the gastrointestinal tract.

gut microflora The bacteria that reside in the intestine, mainly the colon, and act as a barrier to harmful microbes becoming established in the gut.

haemoglobin A protein containing iron, responsible for transporting oxygen in the bloodstream.

haemorrhoids (piles) Swollen veins in the area of the anus which bleed easily and are often painful (similar to varicose veins in the legs).

Harvey and Bradshaw index Modified simple measurement of disease activity in Crohn's disease measured over a 24-hour period.

hepatic flexure The portion of the colon at which the ascending and the transverse colon meet, below the liver.

heredity The transmission of characteristics from parent to child.

histology The examination of tissues under the microscope to assist diagnosis.

hypoalbuminaemia Decreased albumin (protein) in the blood.

hypokalaemia Decreased potassium in the blood.

ileo-anal anastomosis The formation of a pouch following colectomy by re-fashioning loops of ileum into a reservoir, making an artificial rectum and joining it to the anus (Park's Pouch).

ileostomy This is when the open end of the healthy ileum is diverted to the surface of the abdomen and secured there to form a new exit for waste matter.

ileum The third and last part of the small intestine after the duodenum and jejunum.

immune system The tissues and organs that protect the body against harmful organisms and other foreign bodies.

inflammation A natural defence mechanism of the body, in which blood rushes to any site of damage or infection leading to reddening, swelling and pain. The area is usually hot to touch.

internal pouch A reservoir formed from the ileum and attached to the rectum following a colectomy.

iritis Painful inflammation of the eyes.

irritable bowel syndrome (IBS) A condition involving recurrent abdominal pain and diarrhoea or constipation, but without inflammation or other signs of damage to the intestines.

jejunum The second part of the small intestine where most absorption of nutrients occurs.

laxative An agent that acts to cause emptying of the bowel. This may be by purging (irritating the lining) or increasing the volume of stool (bulking).

lesion A term used to describe any structural abnormality in the body.

leucocytes White cells in the blood that help fight infection.

leucocytosis An increase in the number of circulating white cells in the blood.

leucopenia A decrease in the amount of circulating white cells in the blood.

mucus A white, slimy lubricant produced by the intestines.

oedema Accumulation (build-up) of excessive amounts of fluid in the tissues resulting in swelling.

osteoporosis Thinning of the bones due to calcium loss. May be caused by long-term use of steroids or low levels of oestrogen.

pancolitis UC affecting the whole colon.

pathogen Harmful organism causing disease.

pathology The study of the cause of disease.

peptides Two or more amino acids joined together to form one larger molecule. Several amino acids so linked form a **polypeptide.**

percutaneous endoscopic gastrostomy (PEG) A means of feeding a patient directly into his or her stomach by inserting a tube through the abdominal wall at endoscopy.

perforation An abnormal opening (hole) in the bowel wall which causes the contents of the bowel to spill into the normally sterile abdominal cavity.

peristalsis Rhythmic muscle contractions that create a wave-like movement of food contents through the alimentary canal.

peritoneum The membrane lining the abdominal cavity.

peritonitis Inflammation of the peritoneum, often due to a perforation.

polyp A protruding growth from a mucous membrane (e.g. colonic polyp – in the colon).

pouchitis Inflammation of an ileo-anal pouch.

prebiotics Food ingredients and supplements that

encourage the growth of beneficial bacteria in the intestine.

primary sclerosing cholangitis A chronic inflammation of the bile ducts.

probiotics 'Living' bacteria that produce health benefits.

proctitis UC that just affects the rectum.

proctocolectomy The removal of the colon, rectum and anal canal.

prophylaxis Treatment to prevent a disease occurring before it has started.

prostaglandin A hormone that may act to protect the lining of the gastrointestinal tract but which in larger amounts may be a factor in causing inflammation.

proximal Further up the bowel towards the mouth.

pus Thick yellowish liquid caused by inflammation comprising dead white cells and bacteria.

pyoderma gangrenosum A type of chronic skin ulceration which sometimes occurs on the limbs of people with IBD.

radiologist The doctor who interprets X-ray pictures to make a diagnosis.

rectum The lower 20cm of the large intestine, above the anus.

relapse Return of disease activity.

remission A lessening of symptoms of the disease and return to good health.

sacroiliitis Inflammation of the bones in the lower back causing stiffness and pain.

sigmoid The portion of the colon shaped like a letter 'S' or 'C' extending from the descending colon to the rectum.

sigmoidoscopy Inspection of the sigmoid colon with an illuminated telescope called a sigmoidoscope.

skip lesions An inflammation occurring in patients with Crohn's disease that is characteristically patchy in distribution, affecting separate areas of the gut and leaving patches of normal tissue in between.

splenic flexure The portion of the colon at which the transverse and the descending colon meet, below the spleen.

steatorrhoea Presence of excess fat in the stools.

stoma A surgically created opening of a hollow organ to the surface of the body, especially of the intestine on to the abdomen.

stools Faeces.

stricture The narrowing of a portion of the bowel.

suppository A bullet-shaped solid medication put into the rectum.

tenesmus Persistent urge to empty the bowel caused by an inflamed rectum.

terminal ileum The last part of the ileum joining the caecum via the ileo-caecal valve.

total parenteral nutrition (TPN) The delivery of a nutrient solution intravenously so that the patient does not have to eat.

toxic megacolon A dilatation (swelling) of the colon which may lead to perforation, usually in a very severe attack of ulcerative colitis or Crohn's disease. Urgent surgery is usually necessary.

transverse colon The portion of bowel between the hepatic and the splenic flexures.

tumour An abnormal growth which may be benign (non-cancerous) or malignant (cancerous).

ulcer A crater-like open sore on the skin or on a mucous membrane.

ulcerative colitis (UC) A form of IBD affecting the colon.

ultrasound Use of high-pitched sound waves to produce pictures of organs on a screen for diagnostic purposes, by passing a transducer with conducting jelly over a specified body cavity (e.g. the abdomen – abdominal ultrasound).

uveitis An inflammation of the middle layer of the eye, which is called the uvea (or uveal tract).

Acknowledgements

The ideas on which this book was based arose from experience with the management of patients in the department of Gastroenterology at Addenbrooke's Hospital, Cambridge, between 1975 and the present. I am particularly indebted to Sister Allison Nightingale, with whom I wrote the original Addenbrooke's guidance for IBD patients, later made available to all at www.crohns.org.uk.

I am equally indebted to the dietitians whose hard work over many years clarified the nutritional treatment of Crohn's disease. These include Sharon Borland, Eoghan Brennan, Vicky Chudleigh, Jo Cotterell, Gillian Kirby, Monina Mullen, Sally Naylor and Tracy Parker, and in particular Alex Riordan, who supervised the East Anglian trial of diet in Crohn's disease, Jenny Woolner, who developed the LOFFLEX diet and worked hard and long to refine it, and Liz Workman, who was part of our team from the very beginning and supervised the first patients tentatively treated this way.

I am also very grateful to my medical colleagues at Addenbrooke's and the Dunn Nutritional Laboratory at Cambridge whose help and support for the development of new treatments for IBD was so vital. These included John Cummings, the late David Dunn, Marinos Elia, Bill Everett, Alan Freeman, Graham Neale, Derek Wight and Philip Wraight. I was very lucky indeed to be able to work with such a distinguished clinical team.

I also had numerous invaluable discussions on IBD with

many research fellows who worked on IBD in our department. These, now all eminent consultants, included Sean Kelly, Dick Dickinson, Steve Middleton, John Crampton, Dominic Reynolds, Keith Dear, Max Pitcher, Phil Roberts and Robert Atkinson.

Current members of the department of gastroenterology at Addenbrooke's have also been of great support. Dunecan Massey kindly supplied the diagram of genetic changes in IBD on page 24 and Jenny Lee – senior gastrointestinal dietitian – provided details of diets in Crohn's disease as currently used at Addenbrooke's hospital. Specialist IBD Sister Fran Bredin advised on successful methods used to help IBD patients to give up smoking.

Finally, I must thank my personal assistant, Sarah Basser, for typing the manuscript and for her unfailing good temper and humour, and my wife, Maureen, who with the rest of my family has supported me through the years of struggling to understand IBD and to help patients control it successfully.

Index

CD denotes Crohn's Disease; UC denotes ulcerative colitis.